RISK-BASED QUALITY MANAGEMENT IN HEALTHCARE ORGANIZATION

A Guide based on ISO 13485 and EU MDR

Dr. Akash Sharma

Ms. Vriti Gamta

Mr. Gaurav Luthra

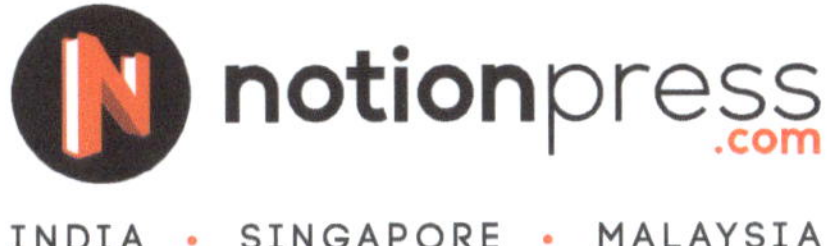

ISBN 979-8-89066-524-9

PREFACE

Welcome to "Risk-Based Quality Management in Healthcare Organization: A Guide based on ISO 13485 and EU MDR." This comprehensive handbook has been meticulously crafted to provide healthcare professionals with the knowledge and practical insights necessary to navigate the intricacies of risk-based quality management in the healthcare industry.

In recent years, the field of healthcare has witnessed significant advancements in medical device technology, leading to improved patient care and outcomes. However, along with these advancements comes the responsibility to ensure the safety and effectiveness of these medical devices. This is where risk-based quality management plays a pivotal role.

ISO 13485, an internationally recognized standard, serves as a cornerstone for quality management in the medical device industry. It provides a framework for organizations to establish and maintain robust quality management systems. Additionally, the European Union Medical Device Regulation (EU MDR) imposes specific regulatory requirements on medical device manufacturers and stakeholders within the European Union. Compliance with these standards and regulations is essential for organizations to demonstrate their commitment to delivering safe and reliable medical devices.

This guide aims to bridge the gap between theory and practice by offering practical guidance on implementing risk-based quality management systems in accordance with ISO 13485 and the EU MDR. It is designed to be an invaluable resource for healthcare professionals involved in various aspects of the medical device lifecycle, including design, development, production, testing, regulatory affairs, and quality assurance.

Within the pages of this guide, you will find a comprehensive exploration of risk-based quality management principles, as well as a detailed breakdown of the requirements outlined in ISO 13485 and the EU MDR. We have endeavored to provide practical examples, case studies, and best practices to illustrate how these principles can be effectively applied in real-world scenarios.

Furthermore, we address common challenges and pitfalls that healthcare professionals may encounter during the implementation of risk-based quality management systems. Our intention is to empower you with strategies and insights to overcome these challenges and ensure successful adoption of these systems within your organization.

It is important to note that this guide does not replace the ISO 13485 standard or the EU MDR. Rather, it serves as a companion to these documents, providing additional context, explanations, and practical guidance specific to risk-based quality management.

We hope that this guide equips you with the knowledge and tools necessary to enhance your understanding of risk-based quality management and its application in the healthcare industry. By mastering these principles and aligning your organization's practices with ISO 13485 and the EU MDR, you will contribute to the delivery of safe and effective medical devices, ultimately improving patient outcomes and fostering trust in the healthcare system.

We extend our gratitude to the healthcare professionals who tirelessly strive for excellence in medical devices. Your dedication to quality and patient safety is the driving force behind the development of this guide. We also acknowledge the contributions of experts, practitioners, and regulatory authorities who have shaped the landscape of risk-based quality management.

We sincerely hope that "Risk-Based Quality Management in Healthcare Organization: A Guide based on ISO 13485 and EU MDR" proves to be a valuable resource on your journey to Risk-Based Quality Management in the healthcare industry.

ABOUT THE AUTHOR

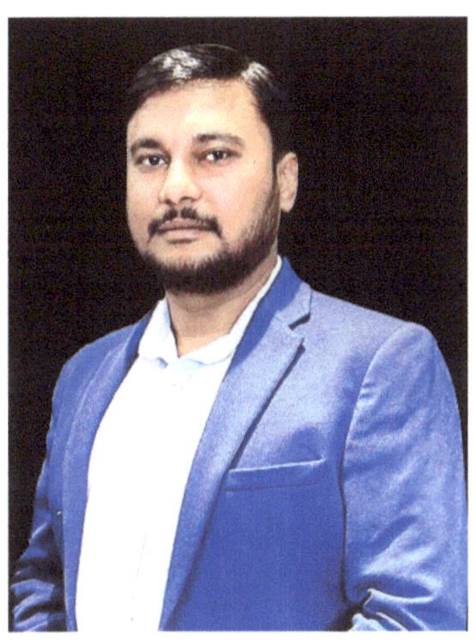

Dr. Akash Sharma is a highly accomplished professional in the field of Regulatory Affairs and Quality Management System for the medical device industry. With a strong academic background and extensive industry experience, Dr. Sharma brings a wealth of knowledge and expertise to the subject of Risk Management in this comprehensive guide. Dr. Sharma holds a Ph.D. & M.Tech in Mechanical Engineering. His research focus has been on the Application of Risk Management Principles in the Medical Device Industry, and he has published over 35 research papers in reputable journals and a book regarding Risk Management in the Healthcare Industry.

Additionally, he has actively participated in more than 15 international conferences, where he has shared his insights and contributed to the advancements in the field. With a career spanning over seven years, Dr. Sharma has gained valuable experience in regulatory affairs and quality management systems. He has a deep understanding of regulatory requirements, particularly in relation to the European Medical Device Regulation (EU MDR), CE certification and ISO 13485 for quality management systems. His expertise also extends to risk management, specifically in accordance with ISO 14971, the internationally recognized standard for managing risks associated with medical devices.

Currently serving as the Regulatory Affairs Manager and Management Representative at KAULMED PRIVATE LIMITED (KAUL-Medizintechnik GmbH), Dr. Sharma plays a vital role in ensuring compliance with regulatory standards and driving quality initiatives within the organization. His hands-on experience in navigating the complexities of regulatory requirements and implementing effective risk management practices makes him a trusted authority in the field.

Dr. Sharma's passion for the medical device industry and his commitment to patient safety and product quality are evident in his work. Through this book, he shares his knowledge, practical insights, and best practices to guide professionals in the medical device industry towards successful risk management practices.

Dr. Akash Sharma's expertise, research contributions, and extensive industry experience make him a valuable resource for professionals seeking to enhance their understanding of risk management in the medical device industry. His dedication to excellence and continuous learning make him a trusted authority in the field.

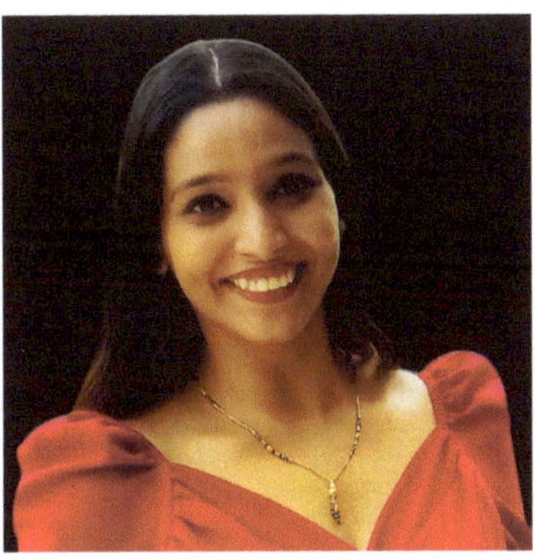

Vriti Gamta is a budding book author with a strong background in the healthcare industry. She holds a Master's degree in Pharmacy with a specialization in Drug Regulatory Affairs (DRA). With over four years of experience in Regulatory Affairs and Quality Management System, Vriti has established herself as an expert in navigating the complex regulatory landscape of the healthcare sector. Vriti's expertise lies in ensuring compliance with regulations and standards related to medical devices and pharmaceutical products. She is particularly knowledgeable in the European Union Medical Device Regulation (EU MDR), which sets out the requirements for placing medical devices on the market within the EU. In addition to her regulatory affairs proficiency, Vriti is well-versed in Quality Management Systems, specifically ISO 13485. This standard outlines the requirements for a comprehensive quality management system for the design, development, production, and distribution of medical devices.

Vriti has also developed a keen understanding of risk management principles, particularly ISO 14971. This international standard provides guidelines for identifying, evaluating, and controlling risks associated with medical devices throughout their lifecycle. Her commitment to advancing knowledge in her field is evident through her publication of a handbook guiding healthcare professionals about Risk Management in Healthcare Industry and seven papers in international journals. These publications showcase her ability to conduct research, analyze data, and contribute to the scientific community within the healthcare industry.

Currently, Vriti holds the position of Regulatory Affairs Executive at KAULMED PRIVATE LIMITED (KAUL-Medizintechnik GmbH), where she plays a crucial role in ensuring regulatory compliance and maintaining high-quality standards for the organization's medical devices and pharmaceutical products.

Vriti Gamta's combination of academic qualifications, extensive experience, and research contributions makes her a respected authority in Regulatory Affairs and Quality Management Systems within the healthcare industry. As a book author, she may reach a larger audience and impart her wisdom and insights, offering invaluable advice to both experts and enthusiasts.

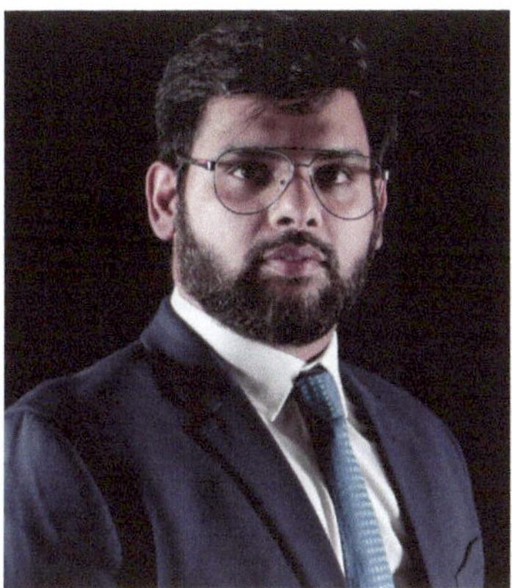

Gaurav Luthra is an accomplished author with a diverse range of experience in the medical device industry. With a career spanning 17 years, he has served as a Managing Director, leading and overseeing operations in the field. His extensive knowledge of manufacturing and new product development, regulatory affairs, quality management systems (QMS), and research and development has positioned him as an expert in his field. Throughout his career, Gaurav Luthra has contributed significantly through his research and publications. He has authored remarkable papers that have been published in renowned international journals.

As a Managing Director at KAULMED PRIVATE LIMITED (KAUL-Medizintechnik GmbH), Gaurav Luthra has been responsible for driving innovation and spearheading research and development efforts within his organization. His focus on new product development has allowed him to stay at the forefront of technological advancements in the medical device industry, ensuring that his company remains competitive and continues to provide cutting-edge solutions. In addition to his expertise in manufacturing and product development. With a holistic approach to his work, Gaurav Luthra emphasizes the importance of quality management systems. He recognizes the significance of maintaining robust processes and procedures to ensure the consistent delivery of safe and effective medical devices. Through his experience, he has implemented and optimized QMS practices to meet the highest industry standards.

Gaurav Luthra's extensive experience and comprehensive understanding of the medical device industry make him an authoritative voice in his field. His dedication to research and development, combined with his expertise in manufacturing, regulatory affairs, and QMS, positions him as a valuable resource for professionals and researchers seeking insights into the medical device industry.

As an author, Gaurav Luthra can communicate complex concepts in a clear and concise manner. Overall, Gaurav Luthra's expertise, experience, and research contributions have solidified his reputation as a prominent figure in the medical device industry. Through his publications and managerial role, he continues to make significant contributions to the advancement and improvement of medical devices, ultimately benefiting patients and healthcare providers alike.

CONTENTS

LIST OF FIGURES

LIST OF TABLES

INTRODUCTION

"Risk-Based Quality Management in Healthcare Organization: A Guide based on ISO 13485 and EU MDR" serves as a helpful resource for healthcare professionals seeking to navigate the complex landscape of risk-based quality management in the context of medical devices. This comprehensive guide offers practical insights and actionable steps to implement robust risk management practices aligned with the internationally recognized ISO 13485 standard and the European Medical Device Regulation (EU MDR).

In today's rapidly evolving healthcare environment, ensuring the safety and efficacy of medical devices is of paramount importance. ISO 13485 provides a framework for organizations involved in the design, manufacturing, and distribution of medical devices to establish and maintain quality management systems. By incorporating risk-based approaches into their operations, healthcare professionals can proactively identify and mitigate potential hazards and vulnerabilities throughout the entire product lifecycle.

The EU MDR, introduced to enhance patient safety and strengthen regulatory oversight within the European Union, places an even greater emphasis on risk management. Medical device manufacturers are now required to conduct comprehensive risk assessments, document risk management activities, and continually monitor and evaluate the performance of their devices in the market. Adhering to the EU MDR enables organizations to demonstrate compliance with rigorous regulatory requirements and gain access to the European market.

Within this context, "Risk-Based Quality Management" equips healthcare professionals with the knowledge and tools necessary to implement effective risk management strategies in line with ISO 13485 and EU MDR. The guide delves into the fundamental principles of risk assessment, control, and mitigation, providing practical guidance on incorporating these principles into daily operations.

From risk identification to risk monitoring, the guide covers a wide range of topics, offering detailed explanations of risk management processes, assessment techniques, and documentation requirements. It also explores the integration of risk management practices with existing quality management systems, emphasizing the synergies between these two critical components of organizational excellence.

Moreover, the guide recognizes the importance of post-market surveillance as an integral part of risk-based quality management. It highlights the significance of monitoring the performance of medical devices in real-world settings, gathering user feedback, and implementing appropriate corrective and preventive actions to address identified risks.

Through insightful case studies and practical examples drawn from the healthcare industry, "Risk-Based Quality Management" illustrates how risk management principles can be applied in various scenarios. This enables healthcare professionals to grasp the practical nuances of risk management implementation and learn from real-world experiences.

Whether you are a medical device manufacturer, regulatory affairs professional, quality assurance specialist, or healthcare practitioner involved in the delivery of safe and effective healthcare services, this guide will empower you to navigate the complexities of risk-based quality management and achieve compliance with ISO 13485 and EU MDR.

With its comprehensive coverage and practical approach, "Risk-Based Quality Management" stands as an indispensable companion for healthcare professionals committed to ensuring the safety, reliability, and quality of medical devices in the dynamic and ever-evolving healthcare landscape.

The Importance Of Risk-based Quality Management In Healthcare

Risk-based quality management plays a vital role in ensuring patient safety, product efficacy, and regulatory compliance in the healthcare industry. Here are some key reasons why risk-based quality management is of paramount importance in healthcare (Figure 1):

1. **Patient Safety:** The primary objective of risk-based quality management is to protect patients from harm. By identifying, assessing, and mitigating risks associated with medical devices, healthcare professionals can minimize the likelihood of adverse

events and ensure patient safety. Through proactive risk management practices, potential hazards and vulnerabilities can be addressed before they pose a threat to patients.

2. **Regulatory Compliance:** Regulatory authorities, such as the Food and Drug Administration (FDA) in the United States and the European Medicines Agency (EMA) in Europe, require healthcare organizations to adhere to stringent quality standards and regulations. Implementing risk-based quality management systems ensures compliance with these regulatory requirements, including ISO 13485 and EU MDR. Compliance not only avoids penalties and legal consequences but also enables organizations to maintain their market access and reputation.

3. **Product Efficacy and Reliability:** A robust risk-based quality management approach enhances the efficacy and reliability of medical devices. By analyzing potential risks, manufacturers and healthcare professionals can optimize device design, manufacturing processes, and performance. This ensures that the products are effective in delivering the intended clinical outcomes and consistently meet the needs and expectations of patients and healthcare providers.

4. **Proactive Risk Identification and Mitigation:** Risk-based quality management encourages a proactive approach to risk identification and mitigation throughout the entire product lifecycle. By systematically assessing risks, organizations can anticipate and address potential issues early on, preventing their escalation and reducing the likelihood of failures or adverse events. This proactive approach leads to improved product performance, reduced costs associated with recalls and corrective actions, and increased customer satisfaction.

5. **Continuous Improvement:** Risk-based quality management promotes a culture of continuous improvement within healthcare organizations. By systematically monitoring and evaluating risks, organizations can identify areas for improvement and implement corrective and preventive actions. This iterative process allows for ongoing optimization of product quality, operational efficiency, and patient safety.

6. **Supply Chain Management:** Risk-based quality management extends beyond the boundaries of an individual healthcare organization. It also encompasses supply chain management, ensuring that risks associated with external suppliers and partners are effectively

assessed and managed. By implementing rigorous quality management practices throughout the supply chain, organizations can minimize the risks of compromised product quality, counterfeit products, and supply disruptions.

7. **Evidence-Based Decision-Making:** Risk-based quality management relies on data-driven decision-making. By collecting and analyzing relevant data, healthcare professionals can make informed decisions regarding risk assessment, risk control measures, and resource allocation. This evidence-based approach enhances the accuracy and reliability of risk management strategies.

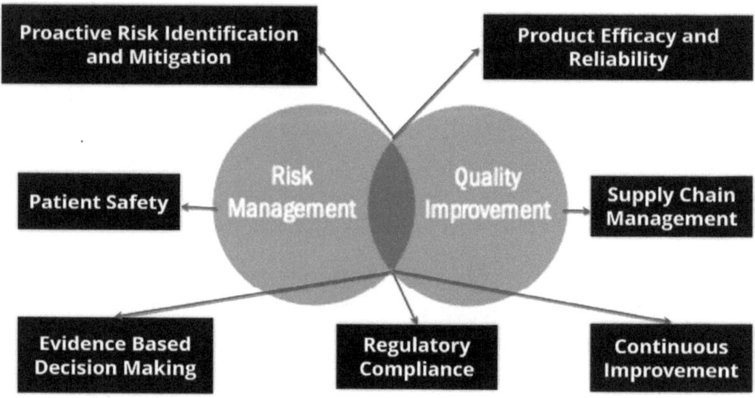

▲ **Figure 1**: Importance of Risk-based Quality Management

Risk-based quality management is crucial in healthcare to ensure patient safety, comply with regulatory requirements, enhance product efficacy, and drive continuous improvement. By implementing robust risk management practices, healthcare organizations can proactively identify and mitigate potential risks, thereby safeguarding patient well-being and fostering a culture of quality and safety throughout the industry.

Overview of ISO 13485 and EU MDR As Regulatory Frameworks

ISO 13485 and the European Medical Device Regulation (EU MDR) are two important regulatory frameworks that govern the quality management systems and safety requirements for medical devices. Here's an overview of each framework (Figure 2):

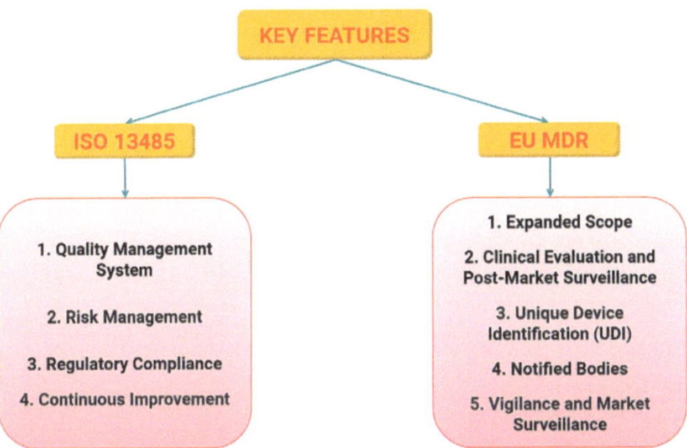

▲ **Figure 2**: Overview of Frameworks

ISO 13485:

ISO 13485 is an internationally recognized standard developed by the International Organization for Standardization (ISO). It provides specific requirements for quality management systems related to the design, development, production, installation, and servicing of medical devices. The standard applies to organizations involved in the entire medical device lifecycle, including manufacturers, suppliers, and service providers.

Key features of ISO 13485 include:

1. **Quality Management System:** ISO 13485 emphasizes the establishment and maintenance of an effective quality management system (QMS) tailored to the unique requirements of the medical device industry. It outlines the essential elements of a QMS, including management responsibility, resource management, product realization, and measurement, analysis, and improvement.

2. **Risk Management:** The standard places a strong emphasis on risk management throughout the product lifecycle. It requires organizations to implement a systematic approach to identify, assess, control, and mitigate risks associated with their medical devices. Risk management activities, such as risk analysis, risk evaluation, and risk control, are essential components of ISO 13485 compliance.

3. **Regulatory Compliance:** ISO 13485 aligns with regulatory requirements in various jurisdictions, including the European Union, the United States, and other countries. Compliance with the standard demonstrates an organization's commitment to meeting applicable regulatory requirements and enhances its ability to market and sell medical devices globally.

4. **Continuous Improvement:** ISO 13485 promotes a culture of continuous improvement within organizations. It requires the establishment of processes for monitoring and measuring product performance, customer satisfaction, and quality objectives. By regularly reviewing performance data and implementing corrective and preventive actions, organizations can drive ongoing improvements in their quality management systems.

European Medical Device Regulation (EU MDR):

The EU MDR is a regulatory framework that governs the safety and performance of medical devices within the European Union (EU). It replaced the previous Medical Device Directive (MDD) and came into effect on May 26, 2021. The EU MDR aims to strengthen patient safety, enhance transparency, and improve regulatory oversight of medical devices.

Key features of the EU MDR include:

1. **Expanded Scope:** The EU MDR expands the scope of regulated medical devices, including certain devices that were previously exempt from regulation. It also introduces a new risk classification system based on the potential risk associated with the device.

2. **Clinical Evaluation and Post-Market Surveillance:** The EU MDR places greater emphasis on clinical evaluation and post-market surveillance of medical devices. It requires manufacturers to provide more robust clinical evidence to demonstrate the safety and performance of their devices. Additionally, manufacturers must establish and maintain post-market surveillance systems to monitor the safety and performance of devices throughout their lifecycle.

3. **Unique Device Identification (UDI):** The EU MDR introduces a UDI system for medical devices, which aims to improve traceability and facilitate post-market surveillance. Manufacturers must assign a unique identifier to each device and provide corresponding product information in a central EU database.

4. **Notified Bodies:** The EU MDR establishes stricter requirements for Notified Bodies, which are responsible for assessing the conformity of medical devices with the regulation. Notified Bodies must undergo a rigorous designation process and have increased responsibilities for ongoing surveillance and market surveillance of devices.

5. **Vigilance and Market Surveillance:** The EU MDR strengthens vigilance and market surveillance activities to ensure the ongoing safety and performance of medical devices. It enhances reporting requirements for adverse events, introduces a new electronic system for incident reporting (EUDAMED), and strengthens the coordination between EU member states in enforcing regulatory compliance.

Objectives and Scope of the Book

The book "Risk-Based Quality Management in Healthcare Organization: A Guide based on ISO 13485 and EU MDR" aims to provide healthcare professionals with a comprehensive and practical resource to effectively implement risk-based quality management systems in the context of medical devices. The book focuses specifically on the requirements outlined in ISO 13485 and the European Medical Device Regulation (EU MDR) and provides guidance on how to align with these regulatory frameworks.

The objectives of the book are:

1. **Understanding Risk-Based Quality Management:** The book aims to provide healthcare professionals with a solid understanding of the principles and concepts of risk-based quality management. It explains the importance of risk management in the medical device industry, the benefits it offers in terms of patient safety and product efficacy, and the regulatory expectations regarding risk management.

2. **Applying ISO 13485 and EU MDR Requirements:** The book guides healthcare professionals in applying the specific requirements of ISO 13485 and EU MDR to their organizations. It breaks down the key elements of these regulatory frameworks, including risk assessment,

risk control, risk mitigation, and post-market surveillance, and provides practical guidance on how to implement them effectively.

3. **Implementing Risk Management Processes:** The book provides step-by-step guidance on implementing risk management processes within healthcare organizations. It covers various aspects such as risk identification techniques, risk analysis methodologies, risk evaluation approaches, and risk control strategies. The aim is to enable healthcare professionals to develop and implement robust risk management practices tailored to their specific organizational context.

4. **Integrating Risk Management with Quality Management Systems:** The book emphasizes the integration of risk management processes with existing quality management systems. It provides insights on how risk-based quality management can be seamlessly integrated into an organization's overall quality framework. This integration ensures that risk management is aligned with other quality-related activities, resulting in a holistic and efficient approach to quality and risk management.

5. **Case Studies and Practical Examples:** The book includes real-world case studies and practical examples from the healthcare industry. These case studies illustrate the application of risk-based quality management principles and provide valuable insights into common challenges and effective strategies for risk management in healthcare settings. By examining these examples, healthcare professionals can gain a deeper understanding of how to apply risk-based quality management concepts in their own organizations.

In a nutshell, the scope of the book encompasses a wide range of topics related to risk-based quality management in the healthcare industry. It covers risk management principles, risk assessment techniques, risk control strategies, risk documentation and reporting requirements, integration with quality management systems, post-market surveillance, and compliance with ISO 13485 and EU MDR. The book is designed to be a practical guide, providing actionable insights and tools that healthcare professionals can directly apply in their day-to-day work to ensure the safety, reliability, and quality of medical devices.

Understanding the Foundations

Understanding the foundations of risk-based quality management is crucial for healthcare professionals to navigate the complex healthcare landscape and ensure the delivery of safe and high-quality care. This chapter provides a comprehensive overview of quality management, risk management, the regulatory landscape, and the integration of risk-based approaches. It sets the stage for subsequent chapters, where more in-depth discussions and practical strategies will be explored to master risk-based quality management in the healthcare industry.

Introduction to Risk-Based Quality Management Principles

Risk-based quality management principles serve as the guiding framework for effectively managing risks and ensuring the quality, safety, and efficacy of medical devices in the healthcare industry, as discussed in Figure 1.1. These principles provide a systematic approach to identify, assess, control, and mitigate risks throughout the entire product lifecycle. Understanding and applying these principles is essential for healthcare professionals seeking to implement robust risk management practices. This section will introduce key risk-based quality management principles:

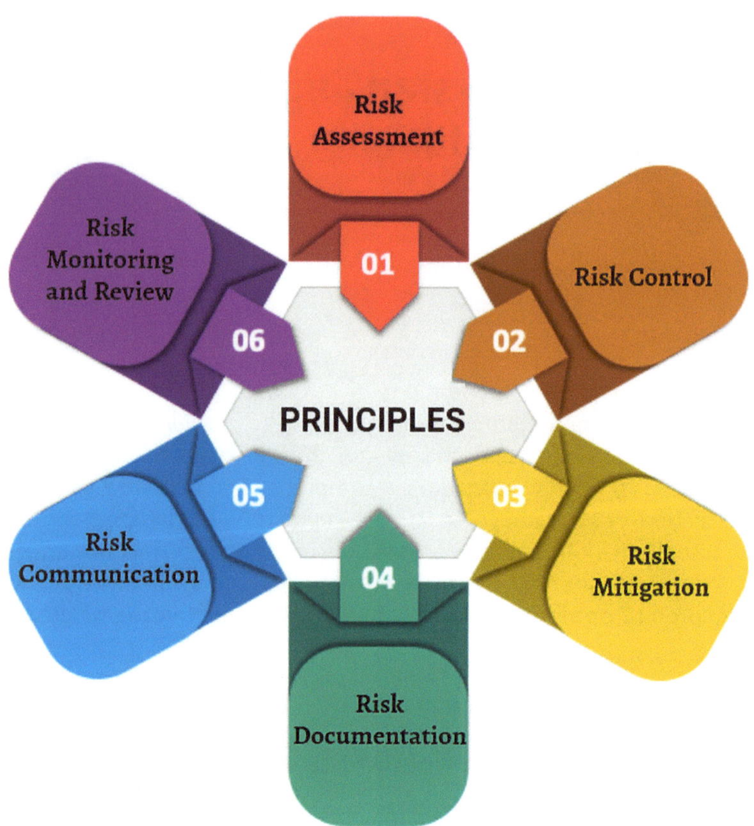

▲ **Figure 1.1**: Principles of Risk-based Quality Management

1. **Risk Assessment:** Risk assessment is the process of identifying and evaluating potential risks associated with medical devices. It involves systematically analyzing the likelihood and severity of harm that may result from identified risks. Risk assessment methodologies, such as FMEA (Failure Mode and Effects Analysis) and PHA (Preliminary Hazard Analysis), are commonly used to systematically evaluate risks and prioritize their management.

2. **Risk Control:** Risk control involves implementing measures to mitigate identified risks. It aims to reduce the likelihood of harm or prevent adverse events from occurring. Risk control strategies may include design improvements, process modifications, use of protective barriers, implementation of safety features, or providing

clear instructions for use. Risk control measures should be based on a thorough understanding of identified risks and their potential impact.

3. **Risk Mitigation:** Risk mitigation refers to actions taken to reduce the severity or consequences of identified risks. It involves developing contingency plans and implementing preventive measures to minimize the impact of risks should they occur. Risk mitigation strategies may include implementing redundancies, establishing emergency response protocols, or conducting regular training and education for healthcare professionals.

4. **Risk Documentation:** Accurate and comprehensive documentation of risk management activities is essential for effective risk-based quality management. Proper documentation ensures transparency, traceability, and accountability throughout the risk management process. This includes documenting risk assessments, risk control measures, risk mitigation plans, and any changes or updates made to the risk management strategy over time.

5. **Risk Communication:** Effective communication of risks is crucial for promoting patient safety and ensuring informed decision-making by healthcare professionals. Risk communication involves conveying relevant risk information to stakeholders, including healthcare providers, patients, regulatory authorities, and other relevant parties. Clear and concise communication enables stakeholders to understand potential risks associated with medical devices and make informed decisions regarding their use.

6. **Risk Monitoring and Review:** Risk-based quality management is an iterative process that requires ongoing monitoring and review of risks. Regular evaluation of risk management processes allows for identification of emerging risks, evaluation of the effectiveness of risk control measures, and implementation of corrective actions as needed. Continuous monitoring and review ensure that risk management strategies remain up-to-date, relevant, and aligned with changing circumstances.

By adhering to these risk-based quality management principles, healthcare professionals can proactively identify, assess, control, and mitigate risks associated with medical devices. This systematic approach helps ensure patient safety, enhance product quality and performance, and meet regulatory requirements. Implementing these principles promotes a culture of quality, safety, and continuous improvement within healthcare organizations.

Overview of ISO 13485 and EU MDR Requirements

ISO 13485 and the European Medical Device Regulation (EU MDR) impose specific requirements on healthcare organizations involved in the design, development, production, and distribution of medical devices. Understanding these requirements is crucial for healthcare professionals to ensure compliance and maintain high standards of quality and safety. Here is an overview of the key requirements of ISO 13485 and EU MDR (Figure 1.2 and 1.3):

ISO 13485 Requirements:

1. **Quality Management System (QMS):**

   ISO 13485 requires the establishment, implementation, and maintenance of a comprehensive quality management system tailored to the medical device industry. The QMS should encompass various processes and procedures to ensure product conformity, traceability, and continuous improvement.

2. **Management Responsibility:**

   The standard emphasizes the active involvement and commitment of top management in ensuring the effectiveness of the quality management system. Management is responsible for defining and communicating the organization's quality policy, establishing quality objectives, allocating resources, and fostering a culture of quality and compliance.

3. **Resource Management:**

   ISO 13485 mandates the allocation of adequate resources, including personnel, infrastructure, and training, to support the effective functioning of the quality management system. Organizations should ensure that employees possess the necessary competence, receive appropriate training, and are aware of their roles and responsibilities.

4. **Product Realization:**

   This requirement focuses on the processes involved in the design, development, and production of medical devices. It encompasses activities such as design and development planning, risk management, design verification and validation, production control, and process validation. Organizations must follow documented procedures and maintain records to demonstrate conformity to these requirements.

5. **Measurement, Analysis, and Improvement:**

   ISO 13485 emphasizes the need for organizations to monitor and measure various aspects of their quality management system. This includes gathering feedback from customers, conducting internal audits, performing management reviews, and implementing corrective and preventive actions. Continuous improvement is a key aspect of ISO 13485, with organizations expected to establish objectives and strive for enhanced performance.

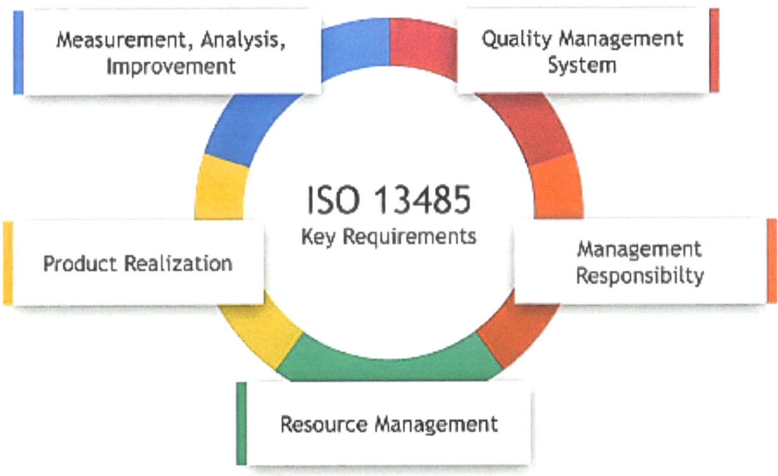

▲ **Figure 1.2**: Key Requirements of ISO 13485

EU MDR Requirements:

1. **Clinical Evaluation and Performance Studies:**

   The EU MDR places greater emphasis on clinical evaluation to demonstrate the safety and performance of medical devices. Manufacturers must conduct a thorough assessment of relevant clinical data and literature and, in some cases, may need to perform clinical investigations or performance studies to support their device's conformity.

2. **Post-Market Surveillance (PMS) and Vigilance:**

   The EU MDR introduces more rigorous requirements for post-market surveillance and vigilance. Manufacturers are obligated to establish and maintain a systematic PMS system to collect proactively and analyze data on the safety, performance, and clinical benefits of their devices. They must also report adverse events, incidents, and field safety corrective actions to the competent authorities and maintain a robust vigilance system.

3. **Unique Device Identification (UDI):**

   Under the EU MDR, medical devices must be assigned a unique device identifier (UDI) to ensure their traceability throughout the supply chain. Manufacturers are responsible for providing UDI information on the device label and registering it in the European Database for Medical Devices (EUDAMED).

4. **Notified Body Involvement:**

   The EU MDR introduces stricter requirements for Notified Bodies, which are independent organizations designated by the competent authorities to assess medical device conformity. Notified Bodies play a crucial role in the conformity assessment process, including issuing certificates, conducting audits, and providing ongoing surveillance of manufacturers' quality management systems.

5. **Economic Operators and Supply Chain Responsibilities:**

   The EU MDR defines roles and responsibilities for economic operators involved in the medical device supply chain, including manufacturers, authorized representatives, importers, and distributors. Each entity has specific obligations related to ensuring device safety, proper documentation, and compliance with the regulation.

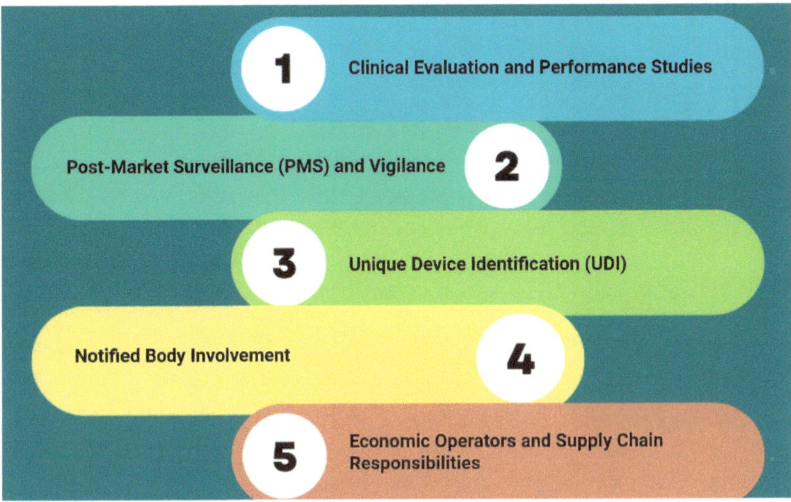

▲ **Figure 1.3**: Key Requirements of EU MDR

These are high-level overviews of the requirements outlined in ISO 13485 and the EU MDR. It is essential for healthcare professionals to consult the official standards and regulations for a comprehensive understanding of all the specific requirements and details applicable to their organizations and products. Compliance with these requirements not only ensures regulatory compliance but also contributes to the overall quality, safety, and reliability of medical devices in the healthcare industry.

Regulatory landscape and compliance considerations in healthcare

The regulatory landscape in healthcare is complex and dynamic, with various regulations and standards in place to ensure patient safety, product quality, and ethical practices. Compliance with these regulations is essential for healthcare organizations to operate legally, maintain public trust, and provide high-quality care. Here are some key aspects of the regulatory landscape and compliance considerations in healthcare (as discussed in Table 1.1 and 1.2):

1. **Government Regulations:**

   Government regulatory bodies, such as the Food and Drug Administration (FDA) in the United States, the European Medicines Agency (EMA) in the European Union, and the National Medical Products Administration (NMPA) in China, establish and enforce regulations for pharmaceuticals, medical devices, and healthcare practices. These regulations cover areas such as product approvals, manufacturing practices, labeling requirements, advertising and promotion, and post-market surveillance.

2. **Quality Management Systems:**

   Healthcare organizations are often required to implement quality management systems (QMS) to ensure compliance with regulations and standards. ISO 9001 is a widely recognized QMS standard applicable to various industries, including healthcare. For medical devices, ISO 13485 specifically addresses quality management requirements. Compliance with QMS standards demonstrates a commitment to quality and helps organizations streamline processes, improve patient outcomes, and mitigate risks.

3. **Data Protection and Privacy:**

   Data protection regulations, such as the General Data Protection Regulation (GDPR) in the EU and the Health Insurance Portability and Accountability Act (HIPAA) in the US, safeguard patient privacy and confidentiality. Healthcare organizations must comply with regulations related to the collection, storage, sharing, and protection of personal health information. This includes implementing data security measures, obtaining patient consent, and providing individuals with rights to access and control their data.

4. **Ethical Considerations:**

   Healthcare professionals and organizations are guided by ethical principles, such as respect for patient autonomy, beneficence, and non-maleficence. Compliance with ethical guidelines, such as those provided by professional medical associations, ensures that healthcare practices uphold integrity, transparency, and patient-centered care. Ethical considerations also encompass issues like informed consent, end-of-life care, research involving human subjects, and conflicts of interest.

5. **Pharmacovigilance and Medical Device Reporting:**

   Healthcare organizations and manufacturers have a responsibility to monitor the safety of pharmaceuticals and medical devices. Pharmacovigilance systems and medical device reporting processes enable the collection, assessment, and reporting of adverse events, product defects, or any safety concerns related to healthcare products. Compliance with pharmacovigilance and reporting requirements helps identify and address potential risks promptly.

6. **Inspections and Audits:**

   Regulatory authorities conduct inspections and audits to ensure compliance with regulations and standards. These inspections may include assessing manufacturing facilities, reviewing documentation, and evaluating quality control processes. Healthcare organizations should be prepared for inspections, maintain accurate records, and address any identified non-compliance through corrective actions.

7. **Continuing Education and Training:**

   Healthcare professionals are required to maintain and update their knowledge and skills through continuing education and training. This ensures compliance with evolving regulations, advances in medical technology, and best practices in patient care. Continuing education programs and professional development activities enable healthcare professionals to stay current and provide the highest level of care.

Below are the two tables highlighting the regulatory landscape and compliance considerations in healthcare, specifically focusing on risk-based quality management and medical device regulations.

▼ **Table 1.1**: Regulatory Landscape

Regulation	Description
ISO 13485	International standard specifying requirements for a quality management system for medical devices. It outlines criteria for organizations to demonstrate their ability to provide safe consistently and effective medical devices.
EU Medical Device Regulation (EU MDR)	Regulatory framework governing medical devices within the European Union. It sets out requirements for placing medical devices on the market, conducting clinical evaluations, and ensuring post-market surveillance.
US Food and Drug Administration (FDA)	The FDA regulates medical devices in the United States. It sets standards and requirements for device safety and effectiveness, including pre-market approval, post-market surveillance, and quality system regulations.
Health Canada Medical Devices Regulations	Canadian regulations governing the sale, importation, and distribution of medical devices. It outlines requirements for device licensing, safety, effectiveness, and post-market surveillance.
Therapeutic Goods Administration (TGA)	Australian regulatory body responsible for the regulation of medical devices. TGA oversees pre-market assessment, conformity assessment, post-market monitoring, and adverse event reporting for medical devices.
Pharmaceuticals and Medical Devices Agency (PMDA)	Regulatory authority in Japan responsible for the approval and regulation of medical devices. It assesses the safety, efficacy, and quality of medical devices, as well as oversees post-market surveillance and inspections.

▼ **Table 1.2**: Compliance Considerations

Compliance Consideration	Description
Risk Management Plan	Develop and implement a comprehensive risk management plan that outlines strategies and processes for identifying, assessing, controlling, and monitoring risks associated with medical devices.
Quality Management System (QMS)	Establish and maintain a robust QMS compliant with relevant regulations and standards, such as ISO 13485, to ensure the effective management of quality and risk throughout the product lifecycle.
Post-Market Surveillance (PMS)	Implement a systematic PMS system to monitor and analyze device performance, gather feedback from users, and report adverse events or incidents to regulatory authorities as required by applicable regulations.
Clinical Evaluation	Conduct thorough clinical evaluations and performance studies to demonstrate the safety, performance, and clinical benefits of medical devices, particularly in compliance with the requirements of the EU MDR.
Unique Device Identification (UDI)	Assign a unique device identifier (UDI) to each medical device to ensure its traceability throughout the supply chain, and comply with the UDI requirements set forth by relevant regulations.
Notified Body Interaction	Collaborate with designated Notified Bodies for conformity assessment, audits, and certification processes, ensuring compliance with their requirements and maintaining regular communication.
Documentation and Recordkeeping	Maintain accurate and up-to-date documentation, including risk assessments, risk control measures, post-market surveillance data, and other relevant records, to demonstrate compliance and facilitate regulatory audits.
Vigilance Reporting	Establish mechanisms for timely reporting of adverse events, incidents, and field safety corrective actions to the appropriate regulatory authorities, adhering to the vigilance reporting requirements specific to each regulatory jurisdiction.

These tables provide an overview of the regulatory landscape and compliance considerations related to risk-based quality management in healthcare. It is important for healthcare professionals to stay updated with the specific requirements and regulations applicable to their respective regions to ensure compliance and promote patient safety.

Compliance with regulatory requirements is crucial to maintain legal and ethical operations in healthcare. It helps protect patient safety, ensure product quality, and foster public confidence in the healthcare system. Healthcare organizations must remain vigilant, stay informed about regulatory updates, and implement robust compliance programs to meet the ever-changing regulatory landscape.

<table><tr><td>Chapter
02</td><td># Risk Management Strategies</td></tr></table>

Effective risk management strategies are essential for healthcare organizations to identify, assess, mitigate, and monitor risks associated with medical devices and patient care (as shown in Figure 2.1). This chapter explores various strategies and approaches that healthcare professionals can employ to manage risks proactively. By implementing robust risk management strategies, healthcare organizations can enhance patient safety, improve product quality, and comply with regulatory requirements.

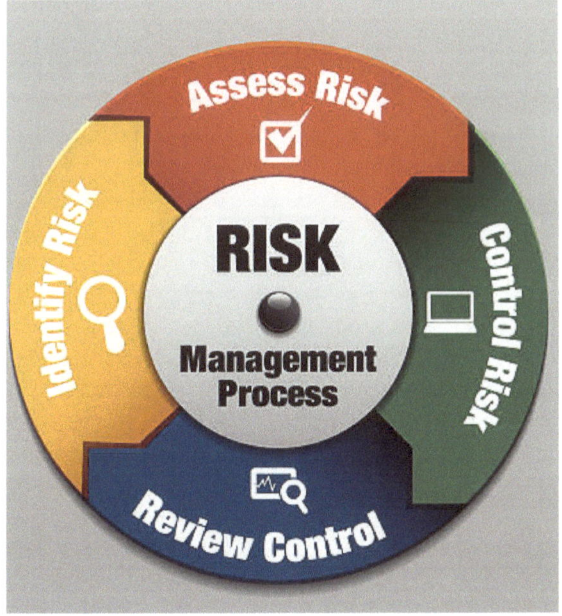

▲ **Figure 2.1**: Risk Management Process

1. **Risk Identification:**

    The first step in risk management is identifying potential risks associated with medical devices and healthcare processes. This involves systematically analyzing the device's design, manufacturing, and use, as well as considering human factors, environmental factors, and potential hazards. Risk identification techniques such as brainstorming, fault tree analysis, and failure mode and effects analysis (FMEA) help capture a comprehensive range of risks.

2. **Risk Assessment:**

    Once risks are identified, they need to be assessed to determine their severity, likelihood, and potential impact. Quantitative and qualitative risk assessment methods can be employed to prioritize risks based on their potential harm. Techniques like risk matrices, risk scoring, and probability analysis aid in assigning risk levels and determining the need for further action.

3. **Risk Control:**

    Risk control measures aim to mitigate or eliminate identified risks to an acceptable level. This involves implementing appropriate strategies and interventions to reduce the probability or severity of harm. Risk control measures can include design modifications, process changes, safety features, training programs, and standard operating procedures. The principle of AFAP (As Far As Possible) guides decision-making in risk control, ensuring that risks are reduced to a level that is reasonably achievable.

4. **Risk Communication:**

    Effective risk communication is vital for ensuring that relevant stakeholders are aware of potential risks associated with medical devices or healthcare processes. This involves transparently sharing information about identified risks, their potential consequences, and the actions taken to control them. Clear communication channels, informative labeling, patient education materials, and healthcare professional training programs facilitate effective risk communication.

5. **Risk Monitoring and Review:**

    Risk management is an ongoing process that requires regular monitoring and review. Healthcare organizations should establish mechanisms to track the effectiveness of risk control measures, collect post-market surveillance data, and conduct periodic risk assessments.

This enables the identification of emerging risks, evaluation of the impact of implemented controls, and implementation of necessary adjustments to the risk management strategies.

6. **Integration of Risk Management with Quality Management Systems:**

Risk-based quality management involves integrating risk management practices with existing quality management systems. Healthcare organizations should ensure that risk management processes are aligned with ISO 13485 and other relevant quality management standards. This integration facilitates a systematic approach to risk identification, assessment, control, and monitoring throughout the organization.

7. **Continuous Improvement:**

Risk management strategies should be subject to continuous improvement efforts. By analyzing data, monitoring outcomes, and gathering feedback, healthcare organizations can identify areas for improvement in their risk management practices. Lessons learned from adverse events, near misses, and customer feedback should be incorporated into the risk management process to drive continuous improvement and enhance patient safety.

Identifying And Categorizing Risks In The Healthcare Industry

Identifying and categorizing risks in the healthcare industry is a critical step in effective risk management. By systematically analyzing potential risks, healthcare organizations can prioritize their efforts, allocate resources, and implement appropriate risk mitigation strategies. Here are some key steps involved in identifying and categorizing risks in the healthcare industry:

1. **Risk Identification:**

The first step is to identify potential risks that may impact patient safety, product quality, or the overall delivery of healthcare services. This can be achieved through various methods, including:

- Reviewing historical data: Analyzing past incidents, adverse events, near misses, and complaints can help identify recurring patterns and potential risks.

- Conducting risk assessments: Engaging multidisciplinary teams, including healthcare professionals, administrators, and risk management experts, to systematically assess potential risks associated with medical devices, clinical processes, and healthcare operations.

- Stakeholder input: Soliciting input from patients, healthcare providers, regulatory authorities, and other relevant stakeholders can provide valuable insights into potential risks and concerns.

2. **Categorizing Risks:**

Once potential risks are identified, they can be categorized into different types or domains to aid in understanding and management. Here are some common categories used in healthcare risk management (as shown in Figure 2.2):

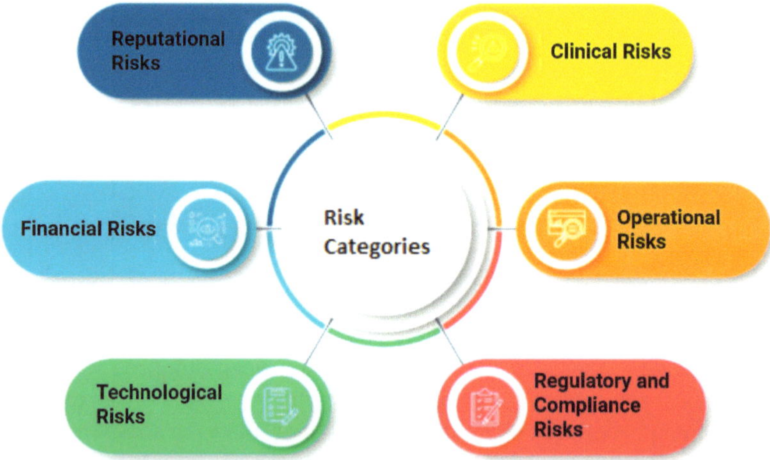

▲ **Figure 2.2**: Categories of Risks

- Clinical Risks: Risks related to patient care and clinical processes, including medication errors, surgical complications, healthcare-associated infections, misdiagnoses, and patient falls.

- Operational Risks: Risks associated with the organization's operational processes, such as supply chain disruptions, equipment failures, facility safety hazards, staffing shortages, and communication breakdowns.

- Regulatory and Compliance Risks: Risks arising from non-compliance with regulations, standards, and legal requirements. This includes risks related to licensing, documentation, data protection, privacy breaches, and violations of healthcare regulations.

- Technological Risks: Risks associated using technology in healthcare, including cybersecurity threats, system failures, data breaches, interoperability issues, and improper use of health information technology.

- Financial Risks: Risks related to financial management, reimbursement challenges, billing errors, fraud, and budget constraints that can impact the organization's financial stability and ability to provide quality care.

- Reputational Risks: Risks that can damage the organization's reputation and public trust, such as media scrutiny, negative patient experiences, malpractice claims, and ethical breaches.

3. **Risk Assessment and Prioritization:**

After categorizing risks, they should be assessed and prioritized based on their likelihood and potential impact. This helps in focusing resources and implementing appropriate risk mitigation strategies. Risk assessment methods, such as qualitative or quantitative assessments, can be used to assign risk levels and prioritize risks for further action.

4. **Risk Documentation and Reporting:**

It is crucial to maintain a comprehensive record of identified risks, their categorization, assessment results, and the organization's response. This documentation supports transparency, facilitates communication, and ensures accountability. Regular reporting on identified risks and mitigation efforts to relevant stakeholders, including management, regulatory authorities, and staff, promotes a culture of risk awareness and encourages proactive risk management.

5. **Continuous Monitoring and Review:**

Risk identification and categorization should be an ongoing process, continually reviewing and updating the risk landscape as new information becomes available. Regular monitoring of identified risks, tracking of risk mitigation efforts, and reviewing the effectiveness of risk control measures are essential to adapt to evolving risks and ensure ongoing patient safety and quality improvement.

By systematically identifying and categorizing risks in the healthcare industry, organizations can proactively manage potential threats and enhance patient safety and overall healthcare delivery. This process enables the implementation of targeted risk mitigation strategies, allocation of resources, and continuous improvement efforts.

Risk Assessment Techniques And Tools

Risk assessment techniques and tools are utilized in the healthcare industry to evaluate systematically and quantify risks associated with medical devices, clinical processes, and healthcare operations. These techniques and tools aid in identifying, analyzing, and prioritizing risks, enabling effective risk management strategies. Here are some commonly used risk assessment techniques and tools in healthcare and summarized in Table 2.1:

1.   Failure Mode and Effects Analysis (FMEA):

FMEA (as shown in Figure 2.3) is a systematic approach used to identify and analyze potential failure modes within a process or system. It involves identifying possible failure modes, assessing their severity, likelihood of occurrence, and detectability. By assigning numerical values to these parameters, a risk priority number (RPN) is calculated, allowing prioritization of risks for further action.

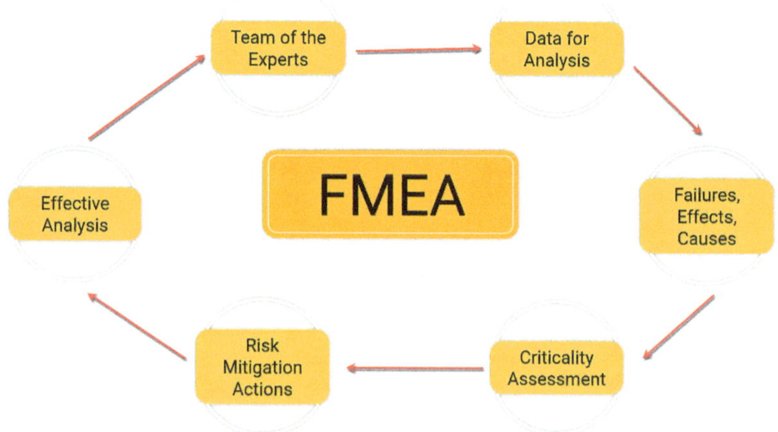

▲ **Figure 2.3**: Overview of FMEA

2. **Hazard Analysis and Critical Control Points (HACCP):**

    HACCP is a preventive risk assessment tool commonly used in the food industry but also applicable to healthcare settings. It identifies and addresses hazards and critical control points in processes to ensure the safety of products or services. HACCP involves conducting a systematic analysis of potential hazards, implementing control measures, monitoring procedures, and establishing corrective actions.

3. **Bowtie Analysis:**

    Bowtie analysis is a visual risk assessment technique that depicts the relationship between potential hazards, causes, and consequences. It utilizes a bowtie-shaped diagram to illustrate the pathways from hazards to potential incidents and the preventive and mitigating controls in place. Bowtie analysis helps in understanding the relationships between hazards, potential events, and risk controls.

4. **Fault Tree Analysis (FTA):**

    FTA is a deductive risk assessment technique that identifies the root causes of a specific event or failure. It uses a graphical representation of a fault tree to analyze the combinations of events or conditions that can lead to the occurrence of an undesired event. FTA helps in understanding the causes and interdependencies of failures and facilitates the identification of risk control measures.

5. **Event Tree Analysis (ETA):**

    ETA is a forward-looking risk assessment technique that assesses the potential consequences and outcomes of an initiating event. It uses a graphical representation of an event tree to analyze the various potential outcomes and their probabilities. ETA helps in understanding the possible consequences of events and aids in the selection of risk mitigation strategies.

6. **Risk Matrices:**

    Risk matrices provide a visual representation of risks based on their severity and likelihood. By categorizing risks into different levels based on predefined scales, such as low, medium, and high, risk matrices allow for easy interpretation and prioritization of risks. Risk matrices help in making informed decisions regarding risk management and resource allocation.

7. Decision Trees:

Decision trees are graphical tools that assist in decision-making under uncertainty. They visually depict different options, potential outcomes, and their probabilities. Decision trees help in evaluating the potential risks and benefits associated with different courses of action, facilitating risk-informed decision-making.

8. Checklists and Questionnaires:

Checklists and questionnaires are simple yet effective tools for risk assessment. They consist of a series of questions or prompts that guide the assessment process and aid in identifying potential risks. Checklists and questionnaires help ensure comprehensive risk coverage and standardize the risk assessment process.

9. Expert Opinion and Expert Panels:

Expert opinion plays a significant role in risk assessment, particularly when dealing with complex or specialized risks. Expert panels or multidisciplinary teams can be formed to gather insights and opinions from subject matter experts. Their expertise helps in identifying, analyzing, and prioritizing risks based on their collective knowledge and experience.

▼ **Table 2.1**: Risk Assessment Techniques and Tools Commonly Used in the Healthcare Industry:

S.No.	Technique	Description	Advantages	Limitations
1	Failure Mode and Effects Analysis (FMEA)	Systematic evaluation of potential failures and their effects	Identifies potential failure points	Time-consuming process
		Identifies potential causes and consequences of failures	Prioritizes risks based on severity and occurrence	Requires multidisciplinary involvement
		Assigns risk scores based on severity, occurrence, and detection	Facilitates proactive risk mitigation	Relies on subjective judgment

S.No.	Technique	Description	Advantages	Limitations
2	Hazard Analysis and Critical Control Points (HACCP)	**Enables early identification of high-risk areas**	**Supports continuous improvement**	**Limited focus on individual process steps**
		Identifies potential hazards in the food manufacturing process	Prevents food-borne illnesses	Primarily used in the food industry
		Evaluates critical control points to prevent, eliminate, or reduce hazards	Focuses on prevention rather than detection	Requires expertise in food safety regulations
		Implements control measures and monitoring procedures	Promotes compliance with food safety standards	Not designed to address all types of risks
3	Fault Tree Analysis (FTA)	**Provides a systematic approach to ensure food safety**	**Enables traceability in the food supply chain**	**Limited applicability outside of food industry**
		Analyzes potential failures and their causes in a logical diagram	Identifies root causes of failures	Complex and requires expertise to develop
		Visualizes the relationships between events and failures	Quantifies the probability of top-level events	Requires extensive data and information
		Facilitates identification of critical events and failure paths	Provides a structured approach for risk analysis	Difficult to update and maintain

Contd…

S.No.	Technique	Description	Advantages	Limitations
4	Bowtie Analysis	**Supports decision-making for risk mitigation strategies**	**Enables systematic investigation of failures**	**Limited focus on human factors and process details**
		Visualizes potential hazards, causes, and consequences	Shows multiple scenarios and their consequences	Relatively new technique in healthcare
		Identifies preventive controls and recovery measures	Helps prioritize risk control efforts	Requires expertise in risk management
		Demonstrates the relationship between causes, events, and outcomes	Enhances communication and understanding	Limited standardized guidance in healthcare
		Supports proactive risk management and incident response	Facilitates continuous improvement efforts	Relies on subjective judgment and interpretation

This table provides a concise overview of the various risk assessment techniques and tools used in the healthcare industry, highlighting their advantages and limitations. It can serve as a quick reference for healthcare professionals to choose the most appropriate technique or tool based on their specific risk management needs.

It's important to note that the selection of the most appropriate risk assessment technique or tool depends on the specific context, scope of assessment, available data, and resources. Often, a combination of techniques may be employed to achieve a comprehensive risk assessment. The chosen techniques and tools should align with the organization's risk management objectives and regulatory requirements to ensure effective risk mitigation and management in healthcare settings.

Prioritizing Risks Based On Severity And Probability

Prioritizing risks based on severity and probability is a fundamental step in risk management. By assessing the potential consequences and likelihood of risks, organizations can allocate resources and implement appropriate risk mitigation strategies. Here's a general approach to prioritizing risks based on severity and probability (as mentioned in Table 2.2 and Figure 2.4)

1. **Define Severity and Probability Criteria:**

    Establish clear criteria for evaluating the severity and probability of risks. This ensures consistency and objectivity in the prioritization process. Define a rating scale or numerical values that reflect the levels of severity and probability.

2. **Assess Severity:**

    Evaluate the potential consequences or impact of each risk on patient safety, product quality, or the organization. Consider factors such as the potential harm to patients, financial impact, regulatory compliance, and reputational damage. Categorize risks into severity levels, such as low, moderate, high, or critical, based on the established criteria.

3. **Assess Probability:**

    Assess the likelihood or probability of each risk occurring. Consider historical data, expert opinions, available research, and the organization's context. Analyze factors such as frequency, historical occurrence, external influences, and internal control measures. Categorize risks into probability levels, such as rare, unlikely, possible, likely, or frequent, based on the established criteria.

4. **Assign Risk Scores:**

    Assign a numerical value or score to each risk based on its severity and probability levels. This can be done using a matrix or a scoring system. For example, a risk matrix can be used, where severity levels are plotted on one axis and probability levels on the other axis. The intersection of the severity and probability levels determines the risk score.

5. Prioritize Risks:

Sort the risks based on their assigned risk scores, from the highest to the lowest. The risks with the highest scores indicate those that require immediate attention and allocation of resources. These high-priority risks pose a significant threat and have the potential for severe consequences with a higher likelihood of occurrence.

6. Determine Risk Response Strategies:

Based on the prioritized risks, develop appropriate risk response strategies. High-priority risks may require immediate action, such as implementing control measures, process improvements, or additional resources. Moderate or low-priority risks may be monitored or addressed through preventive measures or contingency plans.

7. Review and Update:

Regularly review and update the risk assessment to reflect changes in the organization, industry, or regulatory requirements. As new information becomes available, re-evaluate the severity and probability of risks and adjust the prioritization as needed.

▼ **Table 2.2**: Acceptability of Risk

Red Zone	Unacceptable	Cannot be accepted, however if risk control measures lead to either AFAP or Broadly acceptable, then risk is acceptable
Yellow Zone	As far as possible (AFAP)	The risk reduced to as far as possible, however, if risk control measures further can ensure keeping the same level over a period of time with further investigation into the existence of risk, then risk may be considered to be acceptable, being as far as possible. The risk is Acceptable with continuous monitoring of the residual risk through PMS Activities
Green Zone	Broadly Acceptable	The risk has been reduced to as far as possible

Probability	5					
	4					
	3					
	2					
	1					
		1	2	3	4	5
	Severity					

	Broadly Accepted
	AFAP (As far as possible)
	Not accepted

▲ **Figure 2.4**: Different Zones for Acceptability of the Risk

It's important to note that the prioritization of risks is a dynamic process and should be periodically reviewed to account for changing circumstances. Different organizations may have their own specific criteria and methods for prioritization, based on their unique context and risk tolerance. The prioritization process should align with the organization's risk management objectives and regulatory requirements to ensure effective risk mitigation and management.

Risk Documentation And Traceability

Risk documentation and traceability are essential aspects of risk management in healthcare. Proper documentation ensures that risks are well-documented, tracked, and managed throughout the organization. It provides a clear record of the risk management process, facilitates communication, and enables traceability of actions taken to mitigate risks. Here's a closer look at risk documentation and traceability:

1. **Risk Register:**

    A risk register serves as a central repository for documenting identified risks. It captures essential information about each risk, including its description, potential consequences, severity, probability, risk score, and risk owner. The risk register should regularly be updated as new risks are identified, assessed, and managed.

2. **Risk Assessment Reports:**

Risk assessment reports document the results of risk assessments, including the methodology used, the identified risks, their severity, probability, and risk scores. These reports provide a comprehensive overview of the assessment process and serve as a reference for decision-making and risk prioritization.

3. **Risk Mitigation Plans:**

Risk mitigation plans outline the strategies and actions to be taken to mitigate identified risks. They describe the specific control measures, risk reduction activities, responsibilities, timelines, and success criteria. Risk mitigation plans provide guidance on how risks will be managed and help ensure that appropriate actions are taken promptly.

4. **Incident and Near-Miss Reports:**

Incident and near-miss reports document actual or potential adverse events, incidents, or near misses related to identified risks. These reports capture details such as the event description, contributing factors, consequences, and any corrective actions taken. Incident and near-miss reports help identify trends, assess the effectiveness of risk controls, and guide further risk management actions.

5. **Change Management Documentation:**

Changes in healthcare processes, systems, or technologies can introduce new risks or affect existing risks. Change management documentation, such as change requests, change impact assessments, and change implementation plans, should include a consideration of potential risks. This ensures that risks associated with changes are identified, assessed, and addressed appropriately.

6. **Risk Communication Records:**

Effective communication is crucial in risk management. Documentation of risk communication efforts, including meeting minutes, email correspondence, training materials, and stakeholder notifications, helps ensure that information regarding risks is shared transparently and consistently. It facilitates traceability of risk communication activities and ensures that relevant stakeholders are well-informed.

7. **Audit Trail:**

   Maintaining an audit trail of risk management activities and decisions is important for traceability. This includes documenting who performed specific risk assessments, the dates of assessments, updates made to risk registers, and any changes in risk mitigation plans. An audit trail provides transparency and accountability, allowing for review and verification of risk management processes.

8. **Documentation Version Control:**

   Maintaining version control of risk documentation is critical to ensure the accuracy and traceability of information. Clearly identifying document versions, dates, and revisions helps avoid confusion and ensures that the most up-to-date information is used for risk management activities.

By documenting risks and their associated activities, healthcare organizations can demonstrate compliance with regulatory requirements, facilitate effective communication, and support continuous improvement efforts. Well-documented risk management processes enhance transparency, accountability, and the ability to track the effectiveness of risk mitigation strategies over time.

Quality System Integration

E ffective quality management is essential in the healthcare industry to ensure patient safety, product quality, and regulatory compliance (Figure 3.1). In this chapter, we will explore the concept of quality system integration and its significance in harmonizing various quality management processes within healthcare organizations. By integrating quality systems, healthcare professionals can streamline operations, enhance efficiency, and achieve a holistic approach to quality management.

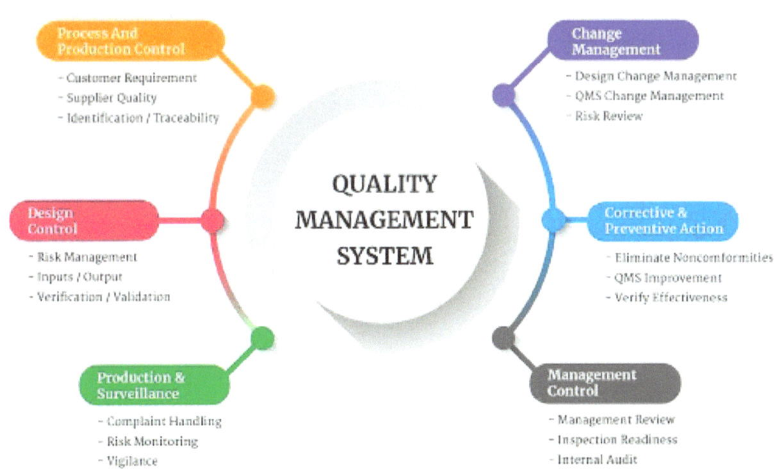

▲ **Figure 3.1**: QMS

Integrating Risk Management Into Existing Quality Management Systems

Integrating risk management into existing quality management systems is essential for healthcare organizations to identify proactively, assess, and mitigate risks that may impact patient safety, product quality, and overall organizational performance. Here are some key considerations for integrating risk management into existing quality management systems:

1. **Assess Current Quality Management System:**

   Start by conducting a comprehensive assessment of your organization's current quality management system. Understand its structure, processes, and documentation to identify areas where risk management can be integrated seamlessly. Evaluate existing quality policies, procedures, and practices to determine their alignment with risk management principles.

2. **Establish Risk Management Framework:**

   Develop a risk management framework that aligns with recognized standards and guidelines, such as ISO 31000:2018. Define clear risk management objectives, roles, and responsibilities within the organization. Establish a risk management policy that outlines the organization's commitment to identifying, assessing, and managing risks throughout its operations.

3. **Identify and Assess Risks:**

   Collaborate with relevant stakeholders, including healthcare professionals, administrators, and risk management experts, to identify and assess risks across the organization. Conduct risk assessments using appropriate tools and techniques such as FMEA, HACCP, or bowtie analysis. Identify potential risks associated with processes, products, equipment, human factors, and external factors. Prioritize risks based on their severity, likelihood, and potential impact.

4. **Integrate Risk Management Processes:**

   Integrate risk management processes into existing quality management systems. This may involve updating quality procedures, work instructions, and templates to include risk management considerations. Ensure that risk management activities, such as risk identification, analysis, evaluation, and mitigation, are clearly defined and integrated into relevant quality processes, such as design controls, supplier management, and change management.

5. **Risk-Based Decision-Making:**

Promote risk-based decision-making within the organization. Incorporate risk assessment results and risk tolerance levels into decision-making processes related to product development, process changes, supplier selection, and resource allocation. Consider risk mitigation strategies when making decisions on quality improvement initiatives or implementing corrective and preventive actions.

6. **Training and Awareness:**

Provide training and education to staff members regarding risk management principles, processes, and tools. Ensure that employees understand their roles and responsibilities in identifying, reporting, and managing risks within their respective areas. Foster a culture of risk awareness and encourage proactive engagement in risk management activities.

7. **Documentation and Reporting:**

Update documentation and reporting systems to reflect the integration of risk management. Develop risk registers, risk assessment reports, and risk mitigation plans that align with existing quality system documentation. Ensure proper traceability of risks, actions taken, and outcomes. Document and report on risk management activities in a transparent and standardized manner to facilitate communication and decision-making processes.

8. **Continuous Improvement:**

Integrate risk management into continuous improvement efforts. Regularly review and evaluate the effectiveness of risk management processes and risk mitigation strategies. Monitor key risk indicators and performance metrics to identify emerging risks or areas for improvement. Use lessons learned from risk management activities to enhance the overall quality management system and drive continuous improvement initiatives.

9. **Regulatory Compliance:**

Ensure that the integrated risk management processes align with applicable regulatory requirements, such as ISO 14971 for medical devices. Stay updated with relevant regulations and guidelines to ensure ongoing compliance. Incorporate regulatory requirements into risk assessments and risk mitigation plans to demonstrate compliance and readiness for regulatory inspections.

10. **Monitoring and Review:**

    Establish a robust monitoring and review process for integrated risk management. Conduct regular audits and assessments to evaluate the effectiveness of the integrated risk management processes. Monitor changes in the external environment, industry trends, and best practices to identify new risks and adjust risk management strategies accordingly.

Aligning Risk-based Approaches With Organizational Goals

Aligning risk-based approaches with organizational goals is crucial to ensure that risk management activities support the overall strategic objectives of the organization (Figure 3.2). Here are some key considerations for aligning risk-based approaches with organizational goals:

1. **Understand Organizational Goals:**

   Gain a clear understanding of the organization's mission, vision, values, and strategic objectives. Identify the key priorities and focus areas that the organization aims to achieve. This understanding provides a foundation for aligning risk management activities with the overarching goals of the organization.

2. **Identify Risks Relevant to Organizational Goals:**

   Identify and assess risks that have the potential to impact the achievement of organizational goals. Analyze the internal and external factors that can affect the organization's ability to meet its objectives. Consider risks related to financial performance, operational efficiency, compliance, reputation, patient safety, and other relevant areas.

3. **Prioritize Risks:**

   Prioritize risks based on their potential impact on organizational goals. Assess the severity and likelihood of each risk and determine their significance in relation to the desired outcomes. Focus on high-priority risks that have a significant potential to hinder the achievement of strategic objectives.

4. **Set Risk Tolerance and Appetite:**

   Define the organization's risk tolerance and risk appetite levels. Risk tolerance represents the acceptable level of risk that the organization is willing to take to achieve its goals. Risk appetite reflects the organization's willingness to pursue opportunities and take calculated risks. Establishing clear risk tolerance and appetite levels helps guide risk management decisions and actions.

5. **Integrate Risk Management into Decision-Making Processes:**

   Integrate risk management considerations into the decision-making processes across the organization. Ensure that risk assessments and mitigation strategies are taken into account when making strategic, operational, and project-related decisions. Assess the potential risks and benefits of various options and select those that align with organizational goals while effectively managing risks.

6. **Define Key Risk Indicators (KRIs):**

   Develop Key Risk Indicators (KRIs) that align with organizational goals. KRIs are metrics or parameters that provide early warning signs of potential risks. Establish specific KRIs that can effectively monitor the risks relevant to the organizational objectives. Regularly monitor and analyze these KRIs to identify emerging risks and take timely actions to mitigate them.

7. **Integrate Risk Management in Performance Management:**

   Incorporate risk management into the performance management framework of the organization. Set performance objectives and targets that include risk management goals. Monitor and evaluate the performance of risk management activities and provide feedback to individuals and teams. Linking risk management performance to overall performance evaluation and rewards can further drive alignment and accountability.

8. **Communicate and Engage Stakeholders:**

   Effective communication and stakeholder engagement are essential for aligning risk-based approaches with organizational goals. Clearly communicate the importance of risk management in achieving strategic objectives. Engage stakeholders at all levels to understand their perspectives and concerns related to risk management. Foster a risk-aware culture where employees actively contribute to risk identification, assessment, and mitigation efforts.

9. **Regularly Review and Adjust:**

   Regularly review and assess the alignment of risk management activities with organizational goals. Monitor the progress of risk mitigation strategies and evaluate their effectiveness. Adjust risk management approaches as needed to ensure ongoing alignment with evolving organizational objectives and external factors.

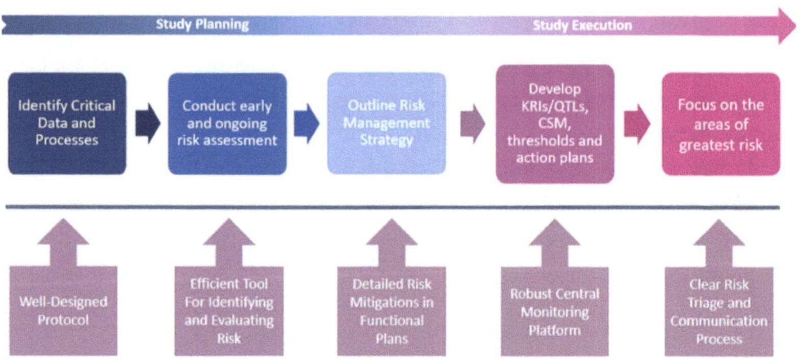

▲ **Figure 3.2**: Aligning Risk-based Approaches

By aligning risk-based approaches with organizational goals, healthcare organizations can ensure that risk management becomes an integral part of decision-making processes and strategic planning. This alignment enhances the organization's ability to identify and manage risks proactively, protect its reputation, improve performance, and achieve long-term success.

Roles And Responsibilities Of Stakeholders In Risk Management

Effective risk management requires the active involvement and collaboration of various stakeholders within an organization. Each stakeholder has unique roles and responsibilities that contribute to the overall risk management process. Here are the key stakeholders and their roles in risk management (as summarized in Table 3.3)

1. **Leadership and Management:**

   Leadership and top management have the primary responsibility for establishing the risk management framework and promoting a risk-aware culture within the organization. Their roles include:

   - Setting the risk management policy, objectives, and overall risk tolerance levels.

   - Allocating resources for risk management activities.

   - Communicating the importance of risk management and promoting its integration into decision-making processes.

   - Monitoring the effectiveness of risk management efforts and ensuring compliance with applicable regulations and standards.

   - Championing continuous improvement in risk management practices.

2. **Risk Management Team:**

   The risk management team comprises professionals who specialize in risk management and play a critical role in implementing risk management activities. Their roles include:

   - Conducting risk assessments, including identifying, analyzing, and evaluating risks.

   - Developing risk mitigation strategies and plans.

   - Facilitating risk management training and awareness programs.

   - Establishing and maintaining risk documentation, such as risk registers, assessment reports, and mitigation plans.

   - Monitoring and reporting on the status of identified risks and mitigation efforts.

   - Collaborating with other departments and stakeholders to integrate risk management into various processes.

3. **Healthcare Professionals:**

   Healthcare professionals, including doctors, nurses, and other clinical staff, have a direct impact on patient safety and the quality of care. Their roles in risk management include:

   - Identifying and reporting potential risks related to patient safety, treatment procedures, medical devices, or medications.

- Adhering to established protocols and guidelines to minimize risks associated with clinical practices.

- Participating in risk assessments and providing input on risk mitigation strategies.

- Communicating and escalating risks to the appropriate channels within the organization.

- Implementing and monitoring risk control measures in their daily activities.

- Participating in training programs to enhance risk awareness and promote a culture of patient safety.

4. **Quality Assurance and Compliance Teams:**

Quality assurance and compliance teams play a crucial role in ensuring adherence to regulations and standards, as well as the organization's quality objectives. Their roles include:

- Integrating risk management into quality management systems and processes.

- Conducting audits and assessments to evaluate the effectiveness of risk management activities.

- Ensuring compliance with applicable regulations and standards related to risk management.

- Reviewing and approving risk documentation, including risk registers, assessment reports, and mitigation plans.

- Providing guidance and support to other departments regarding risk management best practices and regulatory requirements.

- Monitoring changes in regulations and standards to ensure ongoing compliance.

5. **Operations and Process Owners:**

Operations and process owners are responsible for managing the day-to-day operations within their respective areas. Their roles include:

- Identifying and assessing operational risks within their processes.

- Implementing risk mitigation measures in their operations to minimize risks.

- Monitoring and reporting on the effectiveness of risk controls.

- Participating in risk management meetings and providing input on risk management strategies.

- Collaborating with the risk management team to ensure the integration of risk management into their processes.

- Engaging employees in risk management activities and promoting a culture of risk awareness.

6. **Suppliers and External Partners:**

Suppliers and external partners also have a role to play in risk management, particularly in the supply chain and collaborative initiatives. Their roles include:

- Providing information and documentation related to the risks associated with their products or services.

- Complying with the organization's risk management requirements and quality standards.

- Collaborating with the organization in identifying and managing risks within the supply chain.

- Participating in risk assessments and providing input on risk mitigation strategies.

- Ensuring the quality and safety of their products or services to minimize risks to the organization.

Effective collaboration and clear communication among these stakeholders are essential for a robust risk management process. Each stakeholder brings unique expertise and insights, contributing to the identification, assessment, mitigation, and monitoring of risks, ultimately promoting a culture of risk awareness and patient safety within the healthcare organization.

Developing Risk Management Procedures And Workflows

Developing risk management procedures and workflows is crucial to ensure a systematic and consistent approach to identifying, assessing, mitigating, and monitoring risks within an organization. Here are the steps involved in developing risk management procedures and workflows:

1. **Define the Scope and Objectives:**

   Clearly define the scope of the risk management procedures and workflows. Determine the objectives of the risk management process, such as enhancing patient safety, improving product quality, or minimizing operational risks. Ensure that the scope and objectives align with the organization's overall risk management strategy and goals.

2. **Identify Key Risk Management Activities:**

   Identify the key activities that need to be performed within the risk management process. These activities may include risk identification, risk assessment, risk mitigation planning, risk monitoring, and risk communication. Determine the sequence of these activities and their interdependencies.

3. **Establish Roles and Responsibilities:**

   Define the roles and responsibilities of individuals or departments involved in the risk management process. This may include the risk management team, healthcare professionals, quality assurance personnel, and other relevant stakeholders. Clearly specify their responsibilities and expectations in each stage of the risk management process.

4. **Develop Risk Assessment Methods and Tools:**

   Select appropriate risk assessment methods and tools that align with the organization's needs and industry best practices. Common risk assessment techniques include Failure Mode and Effects Analysis (FMEA), Hazard Analysis and Critical Control Points (HACCP), and fault tree analysis. Develop guidelines or templates to facilitate the consistent application of these methods.

5. **Determine Risk Criteria:**

   Establish criteria for evaluating and prioritizing risks. Define the parameters for assessing risk severity, probability, detectability, and other relevant factors. These criteria will help determine the significance of each risk and prioritize them for mitigation efforts.

6. **Define Risk Mitigation Strategies:**

   Develop a framework for selecting and implementing risk mitigation strategies. This may involve identifying and evaluating various options to reduce or control risks. Consider strategies such as risk avoidance, risk transfer, risk reduction through process changes, or the implementation of safeguards and controls. Document the selected strategies and associated action plans.

7. **Establish Risk Monitoring and Review Procedures:**

   Define procedures for monitoring and reviewing risks on an ongoing basis. Determine how risks will be monitored, including the frequency of monitoring and the methods for capturing relevant data. Establish triggers or thresholds that will prompt reassessment or adjustment of risk mitigation strategies. Schedule regular reviews of the effectiveness of risk controls and make necessary updates based on the findings.

8. **Document Procedures and Workflows:**

   Document the risk management procedures and workflows in a clear and concise manner. Include step-by-step instructions, forms, templates, and guidelines as needed. Ensure that the documentation aligns with regulatory requirements and industry standards.

9. **Communicate and Train:**

   Communicate the risk management procedures and workflows to all relevant stakeholders within the organization. Provide training and education on the use of risk management tools, methods, and procedures. Promote awareness of the importance of risk management and the roles and responsibilities of individual involved.

10. **Continuously Improve:**

    Establish a mechanism for continuous improvement of the risk management procedures and workflows. Encourage feedback from stakeholders and incorporate lessons learned from risk management activities. Regularly review and update the procedures and workflows to reflect changes in regulations, industry best practices, and organizational needs.

By following these steps, organizations can develop effective risk management procedures and workflows that facilitate consistent and proactive management of risks throughout the organization. This systematic approach enhances patient safety, improves product quality, and contributes to the overall success and sustainability of the organization.

Compliance Excellence

Compliance excellence is a critical aspect of risk-based quality management in the healthcare industry. Regulatory requirements, standards, and guidelines play a significant role in ensuring patient safety, product quality, and the overall effectiveness of healthcare organizations. This chapter explores the importance of compliance, strategies for achieving compliance excellence, and the integration of compliance with risk management practices. Figure 4.1 shows the questions for Effective Compliance and Figure 4.2 shows the necessity of the same.

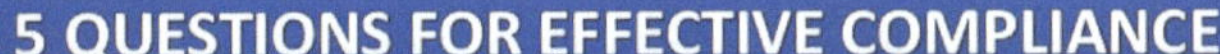

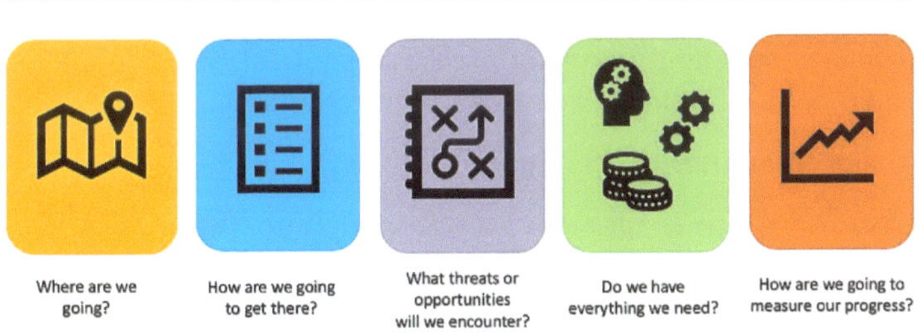

▲ **Figure 4.1**: Effective Compliance

Understanding ISO 13485 and EU MDR compliance requirements

ISO 13485 and the European Medical Device Regulation (EU MDR) are two key regulatory frameworks that govern the quality management systems and compliance requirements for medical devices. Understanding their compliance requirements is essential for healthcare professionals in the medical device industry. Here is an overview of ISO 13485 and EU MDR compliance requirements:

ISO 13485:

ISO 13485 is an international standard specifically designed for medical device manufacturers. It sets out the requirements for a quality management system (QMS) that demonstrates the organization's ability to consistently design, develop, produce, and provide medical devices and related services that meet customer and regulatory requirements. The key compliance requirements of ISO 13485 include:

1. **QMS Documentation:**

   Establishing and maintaining documented procedures and records for all aspects of the quality management system. This includes quality manuals, standard operating procedures (SOPs), work instructions, and records of training, audits, and corrective actions.

2. **Management Responsibility:**

   Ensuring top management's commitment to the QMS, defining quality policy and objectives, establishing a quality management system structure, and providing necessary resources for its effective implementation. Management must also conduct management reviews to assess the QMS's continuing suitability and effectiveness.

3. **Resource Management:**

   Ensuring the availability of competent personnel, adequate infrastructure, suitable work environments, and appropriate monitoring and measuring equipment to support the QMS.

4. **Product Realization:**

   Implementing processes for product design and development, purchasing and supplier control, production and service provision, and product identification and traceability. This includes establishing procedures for risk management, validation and verification, and control of non-conforming products.

5. **Measurement, Analysis, and Improvement:**

    Implementing processes for monitoring, measurement, and analysis of QMS performance, customer satisfaction, and product conformity. Establishing procedures for internal audits, corrective and preventive actions, and continual improvement.

EU MDR:

The European Medical Device Regulation (EU MDR) is a comprehensive regulation that applies to the European Union (EU) member states and governs the safety and performance of medical devices. The EU MDR replaced the previous Medical Device Directive (MDD) and introduces more stringent requirements for manufacturers. The key compliance requirements of EU MDR include:

1. **Device Classification:**

    Classifying medical devices according to their risk levels, ranging from low-risk (Class I) to high-risk (Class III). Manufacturers must ensure conformity with the applicable conformity assessment procedures based on the device classification.

2. **Clinical Evaluation and Clinical Investigations:**

    Conducting clinical evaluations to assess the safety and performance of the device based on clinical data and relevant scientific literature. For certain devices, clinical investigations may be required to generate additional clinical evidence.

3. **Post-Market Surveillance:**

    Establishing post-market surveillance systems to monitor the performance, safety, and risk-benefit ratio of devices placed on the market. This includes implementing procedures for collecting and analyzing post-market data, managing complaints, and conducting periodic safety updates.

4. **Quality Management System:**

    Complying with the requirements of ISO 13485 as a harmonized standard under the EU MDR. Manufacturers must implement a QMS that covers all aspects of device design, development, manufacturing, and post-market activities.

5. **Unique Device Identification (UDI):**

Assigning a Unique Device Identifier (UDI) to each medical device to enhance traceability and facilitate post-market monitoring. The UDI must be provided on the device label and associated with the device's relevant information in a European database.

6. **Economic Operators and Supply Chain:**

Defining the roles and responsibilities of economic operators, including manufacturers, authorized representatives, importers, and distributors, in ensuring compliance with the EU MDR requirements. This includes verifying the conformity of devices, maintaining technical documentation, and reporting adverse events.

It's important for healthcare professionals and medical device manufacturers to stay updated with the latest versions of ISO 13485 and the EU MDR, as well as any additional guidance documents provided by regulatory authorities. Compliance with these requirements demonstrates the organization's commitment to patient safety, product quality, and regulatory compliance in the medical device industry.

Establishing A Compliance Framework

Establishing a compliance framework is essential for healthcare organizations to ensure adherence to regulatory requirements, standards, and guidelines. A compliance framework provides a structured approach to managing compliance activities and mitigating risks. Here are the key steps involved in establishing a compliance framework:

1. **Define Compliance Objectives:**

Identify the specific compliance objectives of the organization. These objectives should align with regulatory requirements, industry standards, and the organization's overall mission and values. Clearly define what compliance means for your organization and what outcomes you aim to achieve.

2. **Identify Applicable Laws and Regulations:**

Determine the relevant laws, regulations, directives, and guidelines that apply to your organization's operations. These may include local, regional, and international regulations specific to healthcare, medical devices, pharmaceuticals, data privacy, and other relevant areas. Stay up to date with changes in regulations to ensure ongoing compliance.

3. **Conduct Compliance Risk Assessment:**

Perform a comprehensive compliance risk assessment to identify potential areas of non-compliance and associated risks. Assess the likelihood and potential impact of non-compliance incidents. Prioritize risks based on severity and likelihood to focus resources on critical areas.

4. **Develop Policies and Procedures:**

Develop a set of policies and procedures that outline the organization's approach to compliance. These documents should address specific compliance requirements, roles and responsibilities, reporting mechanisms, and the consequences of non-compliance. Ensure that the policies and procedures are clear, accessible, and regularly reviewed and updated.

5. **Establish Compliance Monitoring and Reporting:**

Implement mechanisms to monitor and report on compliance activities. This may involve regular audits, inspections, self-assessments, and monitoring of key performance indicators (KPIs) related to compliance. Develop reporting channels for employees to raise compliance concerns and ensure they are aware of the reporting mechanisms.

6. **Training and Education:**

Provide training and education programs to enhance employees' understanding of compliance requirements. Conduct regular training sessions to ensure employees are aware of their roles and responsibilities in maintaining compliance. Offer specialized training for compliance officers and personnel involved in compliance-related activities.

7. **Implement Internal Controls:**

Establish internal controls to ensure compliance with applicable laws, regulations, and internal policies. This may involve implementing segregation of duties, implementing checks and balances, and conducting periodic reviews of processes and systems. Implement controls to mitigate identified compliance risks and ensure ongoing monitoring of their effectiveness.

8. **Conduct Regular Compliance Audits:**

Conduct regular compliance audits to assess the effectiveness of the compliance framework and identify areas for improvement. Audits can be conducted internally or by external experts. Develop an audit plan, define audit criteria, and conduct thorough assessments of compliance practices and processes.

9. **Continuous Improvement:**

Promote a culture of continuous improvement in compliance. Regularly review and update policies, procedures, and controls based on changes in regulations or identified areas for improvement. Encourage feedback from employees and stakeholders to identify potential compliance gaps and implement corrective actions.

10. **Documentation and Record-Keeping:**

Maintain comprehensive documentation and records of compliance activities. This includes documenting policies, procedures, training materials, audit reports, and any remedial actions taken. Proper record-keeping demonstrates a commitment to transparency and accountability.

By following these steps, healthcare organizations can establish a robust compliance framework that promotes adherence to regulatory requirements, mitigates compliance risks, and fosters a culture of compliance throughout the organization.

Document Control And Recordkeeping For Compliance

Document control and recordkeeping play a crucial role in compliance management within healthcare organizations. Effective document control ensures that the most current and accurate versions of documents are accessible to relevant personnel, while recordkeeping enables the organization to maintain a comprehensive and auditable history of compliance-related activities. Here are key considerations for document control and recordkeeping for compliance:

Document Control:

1. **Document Identification and Version Control:**

   Assign unique identifiers (e.g., document numbers or codes) to each document to ensure easy identification. Implement version control mechanisms to manage document revisions, including version numbers, revision dates, and tracking changes made to the document.

2. **Document Approval and Review:**

   Establish a process for document approval and review. Designate responsible individuals or departments for reviewing and approving documents to ensure accuracy, relevance, and compliance with regulatory requirements. Maintain records of document approvals and reviews.

3. **Document Distribution and Access:**

   Implement controls to ensure that documents are distributed only to authorized individuals. Define access levels and permissions based on job roles and responsibilities. Utilize document management systems or intranets to facilitate secure and controlled access to documents.

4. **Document Retention and Archiving:**

   Define the retention periods for different types of documents based on regulatory requirements and organizational needs. Establish protocols for archiving and retrieving documents, ensuring they are stored securely and are easily accessible when needed.

5. **Document Change Control:**

    Implement a change control process to manage modifications to documents. Require appropriate approvals and notifications for document changes. Track and document the reasons for changes and ensure all affected parties are notified of the changes.

Recordkeeping:

1. **Record Identification and Classification:**

    Establish a system for identifying and classifying records based on their type and relevance to compliance. Develop a record classification scheme that aligns with regulatory requirements and organizational needs.

2. **Record Retention and Storage:**

    Define the retention periods for different types of records. Store records securely, ensuring they are protected from unauthorized access, loss, damage, or tampering. Implement backup and disaster recovery measures to safeguard records.

3. **Record Indexing and Organization:**

    Develop an indexing system to facilitate easy retrieval and organization of records. Use consistent naming conventions and metadata to categorize records. Implement logical folder structures and electronic search capabilities to streamline record management.

4. **Record Access and Security:**

    Control access to records to ensure confidentiality, integrity, and availability. Define access levels and permissions based on job roles and responsibilities. Implement audit trails to track record access and modifications.

5. **Record Retention Schedule and Disposal:**

    Adhere to a record retention schedule that aligns with regulatory requirements. Regularly review and update the retention schedule based on changes in regulations. Establish protocols for the secure disposal of records at the end of their retention period.

6.   **Record Preservation and Auditability:**

Maintain records in a manner that preserves their integrity and authenticity. Implement measures to prevent unauthorized alterations or deletions. Ensure that records are auditable and can be presented as evidence of compliance activities when required.

Regularly review and update document control and recordkeeping processes to adapt to changes in regulatory requirements and organizational needs. Conduct internal audits to assess the effectiveness of document control and recordkeeping practices and implement corrective actions as necessary.

Conducting Internal Audits And Addressing Non-conformities

Conducting internal audits and addressing non-conformities are critical components of an effective compliance management system. Internal audits help assess the organization's compliance with regulatory requirements, internal policies, and industry standards. Addressing non-conformities identified during audits ensures that corrective actions are taken to rectify compliance gaps and mitigate risks. Here are the key steps involved in conducting internal audits and addressing non-conformities:

1.   **Audit Planning:**

Define the scope and objectives of the internal audit. Identify the compliance areas, processes, or departments to be audited based on their risk profile and regulatory importance. Develop an audit plan that includes the audit schedule, criteria, and resources required for the audit.

2.   **Conducting the Audit:**

Perform the audit activities according to the defined plan. This involves gathering relevant information, conducting interviews and observations, reviewing documents and records, and assessing compliance against established criteria, such as regulatory requirements, policies, and industry standards. Use appropriate audit techniques, such as sampling, to ensure a comprehensive evaluation.

3. **Non-Conformity Identification:**

During the audit, identify non-conformities, which are instances where the organization fails to comply with regulatory requirements, internal policies, or industry standards. Document these non-conformities, providing clear descriptions and supporting evidence. Non-conformities can include deviations from procedures, incomplete documentation, lack of training, or any other identified compliance gaps.

4. **Non-Conformity Classification and Prioritization:**

Classify non-conformities based on their severity, potential impact, and frequency. Prioritize them according to the level of risk they pose to the organization and patient safety. This allows for a focused approach in addressing the most critical non-conformities first.

5. **Corrective and Preventive Actions (CAPA):**

Develop a Corrective and Preventive Action (CAPA) plan to address each identified non-conformity. Corrective actions aim to resolve the immediate non-conformity and prevent its recurrence, while preventive actions aim to eliminate the root cause to prevent similar non-conformities in the future. Assign responsibility for each CAPA, set deadlines, and establish a follow-up process to monitor the completion of actions.

6. **Implementation of CAPAs:**

Implement the identified CAPAs within the specified timeframe. This may involve process improvements, additional training, policy revisions, or changes to procedures or systems. Ensure that all relevant stakeholders are informed of the CAPAs and their responsibilities in implementing them effectively.

7. **Verification and Effectiveness:**

Verify the effectiveness of the implemented CAPAs through objective evidence. This can include conducting follow-up audits, reviewing updated documentation, and analyzing process performance data. Assess whether the actions taken have effectively addressed the non-conformities and improved compliance.

8. **Documentation and Reporting:**

    Document all audit findings, non-conformities, and CAPAs in a clear and comprehensive manner. Maintain accurate records of the audit process, including the audit plan, audit reports, and evidence of CAPA completion. Report the audit results to relevant stakeholders, such as management, compliance officers, and regulatory authorities, as required.

9. **Continuous Improvement:**

    Use the audit findings and lessons learned to drive continuous improvement. Analyze recurring non-conformities and identify trends or systemic issues that may require broader process improvements or policy changes. Update procedures, provide additional training, and enhance controls to prevent non-conformities in the future.

By following these steps, healthcare organizations can effectively conduct internal audits, identify non-conformities, and implement appropriate corrective and preventive actions to improve compliance and mitigate risks. This ensures ongoing compliance with regulatory requirements, enhances patient safety, and supports the organization's commitment to quality and excellence.

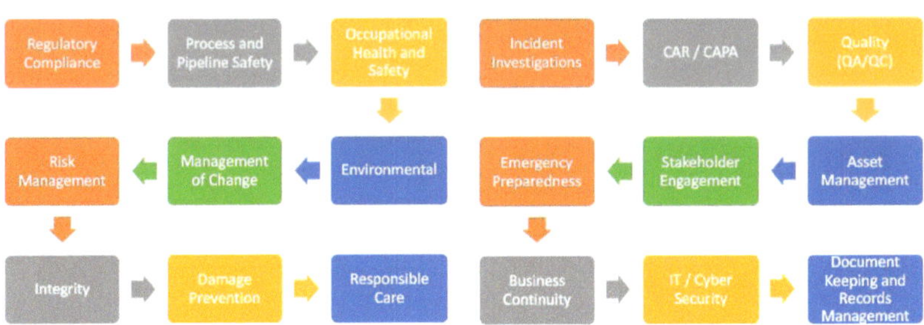

▲ **Figure 4.2**: Why Effective Compliance is Necessary?

Risk Mitigation Techniques

In this chapter, we will explore various risk mitigation techniques that healthcare organizations can employ to minimize the impact of identified risks. Risk mitigation is a proactive approach aimed at reducing the likelihood and severity of potential risks. By implementing effective mitigation strategies, organizations can safeguard patient safety, enhance product quality, and maintain regulatory compliance. This chapter will cover a range of techniques and best practices for risk mitigation in the healthcare industry.

RISK MITIGATION PLAN

Steps to Creating a Risk Mitigation Plan

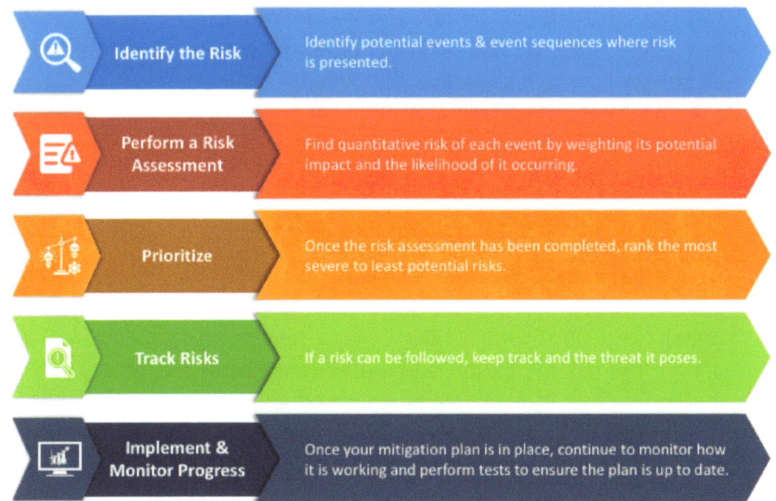

▲ **Figure 5.1**: Risk Mitigation Plan

Implementing Risk Mitigation Strategies In Healthcare Settings

Implementing risk mitigation strategies in healthcare settings is crucial to minimize potential risks and ensure patient safety. Here are some key steps to implement risk mitigation strategies effectively:

1. **Identify and Assess Risks:** Conduct a thorough risk assessment to identify potential risks within the healthcare setting. This may include analyzing processes, equipment, human factors, and environmental factors. Prioritize risks based on their severity, likelihood, and potential impact on patient safety and organizational goals.

2. **Develop Risk Mitigation Plans:** Once risks are identified, develop comprehensive risk mitigation plans. Each plan should outline specific strategies, actions, and control measures to reduce or eliminate the identified risks. Engage relevant stakeholders, including healthcare professionals, administrators, and risk management teams, to ensure a collaborative approach.

3. **Implement Risk Controls:** Put risk controls into action based on the identified mitigation strategies. This may involve implementing safety protocols, improving equipment maintenance processes, enhancing training and education programs, or modifying workflows and procedures. Ensure that risk controls are properly communicated, understood, and followed by all relevant personnel.

4. **Monitor and Evaluate:** Continuously monitor the effectiveness of implemented risk mitigation strategies. Establish monitoring mechanisms, such as regular inspections, audits, and data analysis, to track the progress and outcomes of risk controls. Evaluate whether the implemented strategies are achieving the desired risk reduction and adjust them as necessary.

5. **Engage and Empower Staff:** Engage healthcare professionals and staff in the risk mitigation process. Foster a culture of safety and risk awareness by providing training and education on risk management principles and practices. Encourage open communication channels for reporting potential risks, incidents, and near misses. Empower staff to actively participate in identifying and implementing risk mitigation strategies.

6. **Regularly Review and Update:** Conduct regular reviews of risk mitigation strategies to ensure their ongoing relevance and effectiveness. Stay updated on industry best practices, regulatory requirements, and advancements in healthcare technology to identify new risks and mitigation opportunities. Update risk mitigation plans and controls accordingly.

7. **Incident Reporting and Analysis:** Establish a robust incident reporting and analysis system to capture and analyze incidents, near misses, and adverse events. Investigate incidents to identify causes and contributing factors. Implement corrective actions to prevent recurrence and continuously improve risk mitigation strategies.

8. **Collaborate with External Partners:** Collaborate with external partners, such as regulatory authorities, industry associations, and healthcare networks, to stay informed about emerging risks and best practices. Engage in knowledge-sharing initiatives, participate in bench-marking exercises, and learn from the experiences of others in the healthcare community.

9. **Document and Communicate:** Document all risk mitigation strategies, controls, and outcomes. Maintain comprehensive records of risk assessments, mitigation plans, incident reports, and corrective actions. Ensure that this information is readily accessible to relevant stakeholders. Communicate the implemented risk mitigation strategies and their importance to staff, patients, and other involved parties.

10. **Continuous Improvement:** Emphasize a culture of continuous improvement in risk mitigation. Encourage feedback, evaluate the effectiveness of risk mitigation efforts, and seek opportunities to optimize processes and enhance patient safety. Regularly review and update risk mitigation strategies based on lessons learned, industry advancements, and changing healthcare landscapes.

By following these steps, healthcare settings can implement effective risk mitigation strategies that enhance patient safety, ensure regulatory compliance, and foster a culture of proactive risk management. Remember, risk mitigation is an ongoing process that requires commitment, collaboration, and continuous improvement to protect the well-being of patients and the organization as a whole.

Process Controls And Validation Protocols

Process controls and validation protocols are essential components of risk-based quality management in healthcare. They help ensure that processes within the healthcare setting are consistently performed in a controlled manner and meet predefined quality standards. Here's an overview of process controls and validation protocols:

Process Controls:

Process controls are measures put in place to monitor, control, and improve the various processes involved in healthcare operations. They aim to minimize process variations, mitigate risks, and ensure the delivery of safe and high-quality healthcare services. Some common types of process controls include (Figure 5.2 and 5.3):

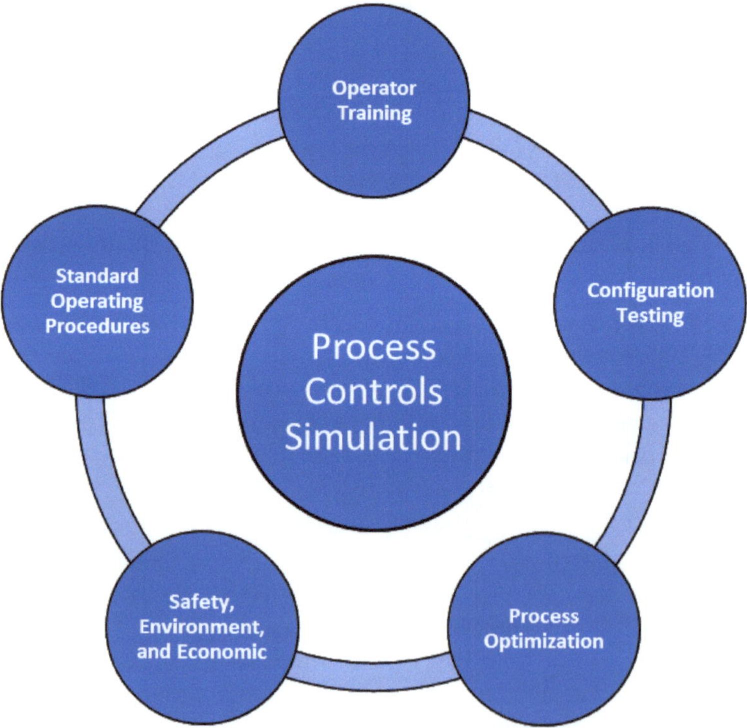

▲ **Figure 5.2**: Simulation for Process Control

1. **Standard Operating Procedures (SOPs):** SOPs provide detailed instructions for carrying out specific tasks or processes. They serve as a guide for healthcare professionals to ensure consistency and adherence to predefined procedures.

2. **Training and Competency Assessment:** Adequate training and competency assessment programs are implemented to ensure that healthcare professionals possess the necessary knowledge and skills to perform their assigned tasks effectively and safely.

3. **Equipment and Instrumentation Controls:** Regular calibration, maintenance, and verification of equipment and instruments are conducted to ensure their accuracy and reliability. Controls may include temperature monitoring, equipment maintenance schedules, and equipment performance validation.

4. **Environmental Controls:** Environmental controls are put in place to maintain appropriate conditions for healthcare operations. This may involve controlling temperature, humidity, air quality, and cleanliness to prevent contamination and ensure patient safety.

5. **Documentation Controls:** Documentation controls involve proper documentation and recordkeeping of processes, activities, and outcomes. This ensures traceability, accountability, and the availability of critical information for audit and regulatory compliance purposes.

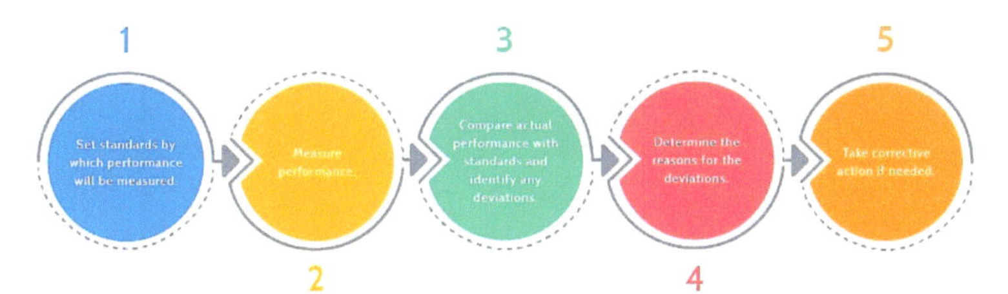

▲ **Figure 5.3**: Overview of Process Control

Validation Protocols:

Validation protocols are systematic procedures used to confirm that processes, equipment, systems, or software perform as intended and meet predefined requirements. They provide evidence that the processes or systems are capable of consistently delivering desired outcomes. Key validation protocols include (Figure 5.4):

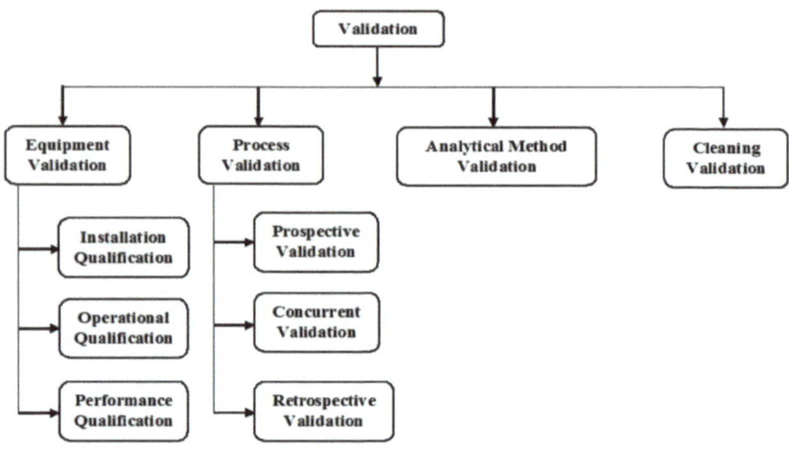

▲ **Figure 5.4**: Types of Validation Protocols

1. **Process Validation:** Process validation ensures that a specific process consistently produces results that meet predetermined quality standards. It involves conducting a series of tests and evaluations to demonstrate the process's capability, stability, and reliability. Process validation is often conducted for critical processes such as sterilization, manufacturing, or laboratory testing.

2. **Equipment Validation:** Equipment validation involves verifying and documenting that equipment performs consistently and reliably within its specified operating parameters. It includes installation qualification (IQ), operational qualification (OQ), and performance qualification (PQ) to ensure that equipment is properly installed, functions correctly, and produces accurate and reliable results.

3. **Cleaning and Sterilization Validation:** Cleaning and sterilization validation protocols are critical for ensuring the effectiveness of cleaning and sterilization processes in eliminating or reducing

microbial contamination. These protocols validate the procedures, parameters, and methods used for cleaning and sterilizing medical devices, instruments, and equipment.

4. **Analytical Method Validation:** Analytical method validation is performed to demonstrate that an analytical method used for testing or analysis produces reliable and accurate results. It involves assessing parameters such as specificity, accuracy, precision, linearity, and robustness.

Validation protocols typically include clear objectives, testing methods, acceptance criteria, and documentation requirements. They are performed during the initial qualification phase and periodically reviewed and updated as necessary to ensure ongoing compliance and process optimization.

By implementing robust process controls and conducting validation protocols, healthcare organizations can ensure that their processes are controlled, validated, and continuously improved. This helps mitigate risks, enhance patient safety, and maintain regulatory compliance throughout healthcare operations.

Post-market Surveillance And Adverse Event Reporting

Post-market surveillance and adverse event reporting play vital roles in ensuring the ongoing safety and effectiveness of medical devices and pharmaceutical products after they have been approved or cleared for marketing. These activities help identify and address any potential risks or issues that may arise once products are used by patients or healthcare professionals. Here's an overview of post-market surveillance and adverse event reporting:

Post-Market Surveillance:

Post-market surveillance refers to the systematic monitoring and evaluation of the performance, safety, and quality of medical devices and pharmaceutical products once they are available on the market. The primary objectives of post-market surveillance include (Figure 5.5):

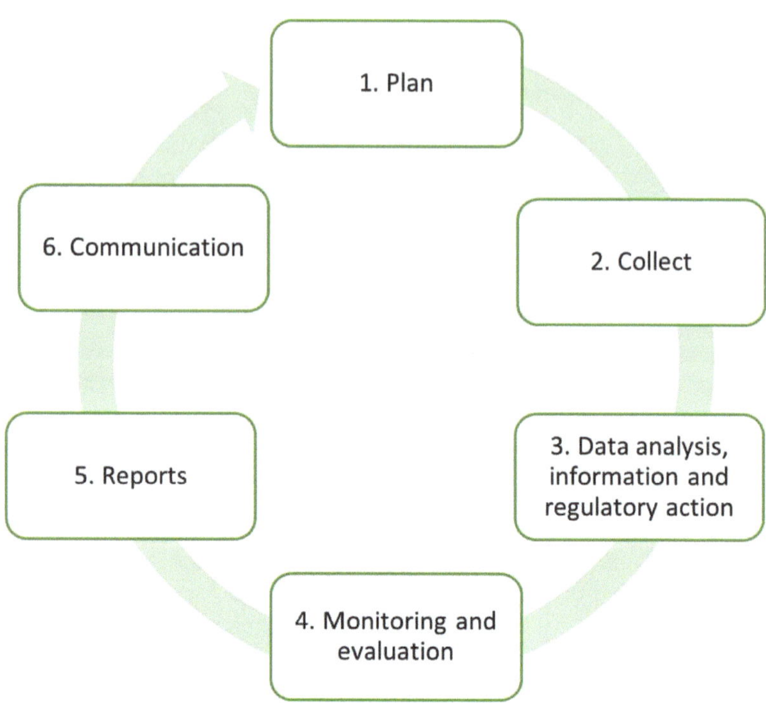

▲ **Figure 5.5**: Post-market Surveillance Activities

1. **Detecting and Investigating Adverse Events:** Post-market surveillance aims to identify and investigate adverse events, which are any undesirable or unintended occurrences associated using a medical device or pharmaceutical product. Adverse events can include device malfunctions, product defects, medication errors, side effects, or any other issues that may cause harm to patients.

2. **Assessing Product Performance:** Post-market surveillance activities help assess the performance of products in real-world conditions. This includes monitoring how products are being used, evaluating their effectiveness, and identifying any potential issues or limitations that may arise during routine use.

3. **Identifying Emerging Risks:** By collecting and analyzing data from various sources, including adverse event reports, clinical studies, registries, and feedback from healthcare professionals and patients, post-market surveillance helps identify emerging risks or trends

associated with specific products or product categories. This information can guide regulatory authorities and manufacturers in taking appropriate actions to mitigate risks.

4. **Evaluating and Updating Risk-Benefit Profile:** Post-market surveillance helps evaluate the overall risk-benefit profile of medical devices and pharmaceutical products. It involves continuously assessing the balance between the potential benefits of a product and any associated risks, taking into account new information and data gathered during post-market surveillance activities.

Adverse Event Reporting:

Adverse event reporting is a critical component of post-market surveillance. It involves the collection, documentation, and reporting of any adverse events or product-related issues encountered by healthcare professionals, patients, or other stakeholders. Key aspects of adverse event reporting include (Figure 5.6):

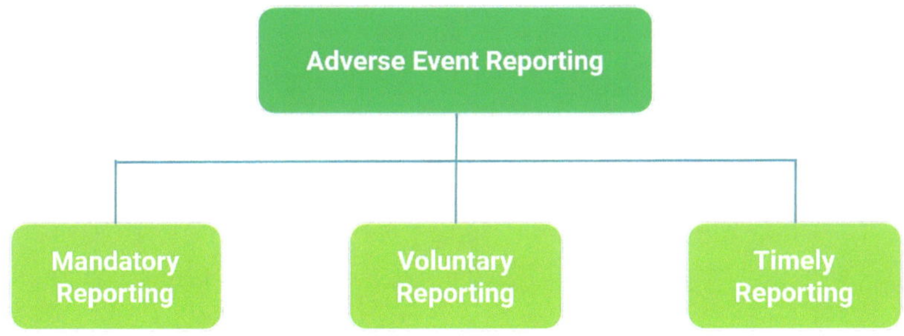

▲ **Figure 5.6**: Types of Adverse Event Reporting

1. **Mandatory Reporting:** Regulatory authorities typically require manufacturers, healthcare professionals, and other relevant parties to report adverse events associated with medical devices and pharmaceutical products. These mandatory reporting requirements ensure that potential risks and safety concerns are promptly communicated to regulatory authorities.

2. **Voluntary Reporting:** Voluntary adverse event reporting allows healthcare professionals, patients, and consumers to report any adverse events they experience or observe. Voluntary reporting systems, such as online reporting portals or hotlines, provide channels for individuals to share their experiences and contribute to the overall safety surveillance of products.

3. **Timely Reporting:** Adverse events should be reported as soon as possible to enable prompt investigation and appropriate actions. Regulatory authorities typically define specific timelines for reporting, depending on the severity and urgency of the event.

4. **Data Collection and Analysis:** Adverse event reports are collected and analyzed to identify patterns, trends, and potential risks associated with specific products. These reports, along with other post-market surveillance data, contribute to ongoing risk assessments and inform decision-making processes.

5. **Follow-up and Corrective Actions:** Regulatory authorities and manufacturers are responsible for conducting thorough investigations of reported adverse events. Based on the findings, appropriate corrective actions may be taken, such as product recalls, labeling updates, safety communications, or modifications to manufacturing processes.

6. **Signal Detection and Risk Communication:** Adverse event reporting data contributes to signal detection, which involves the identification of new or emerging safety concerns related to specific products. Regulatory authorities use this information to issue safety alerts, updated warnings, or guidance to healthcare professionals and patients, ensuring that potential risks are communicated effectively.

Post-market surveillance and adverse event reporting serve as important feedback mechanisms to monitor product safety continuously and make informed decisions regarding regulatory requirements, product modifications, and risk management strategies. These activities promote patient safety and enable regulatory authorities and manufacturers to take proactive measures to address potential risks and ensure the ongoing quality and effectiveness of healthcare products.

Supplier Qualification And Control

Supplier qualification and control are critical aspects of risk-based quality management in healthcare. They involve assessing, selecting, and managing suppliers to ensure that they meet the necessary quality standards and regulatory requirements. Here's an overview of supplier qualification and control:

Supplier Qualification:

Supplier qualification is the process of evaluating and assessing potential suppliers to determine their capability to meet quality requirements and deliver products or services that meet the organization's needs. Key steps in the supplier qualification process include (Figure 5.7):

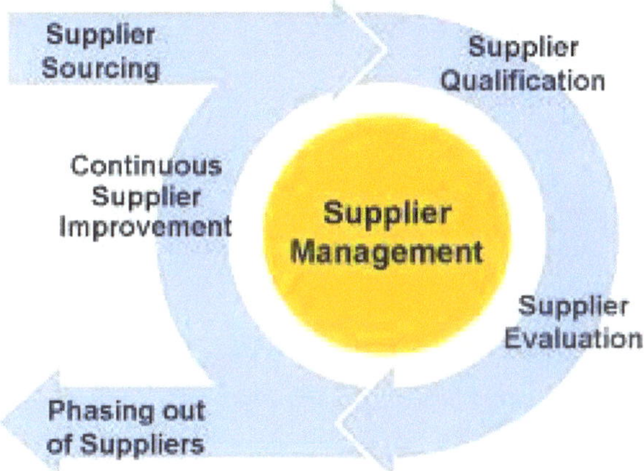

▲ **Figure 5.7**: Supplier Qualification and Control

1. **Define Supplier Requirements:** Clearly define the requirements and criteria that suppliers must meet, including quality standards, regulatory compliance, product specifications, delivery timelines, and other relevant factors.

2. **Supplier Assessment:** Conduct a comprehensive evaluation of potential suppliers to assess their capabilities, quality management systems, manufacturing processes, track record, financial stability, and overall suitability to meet the organization's needs.

3. **Audit and Inspection:** Perform on-site audits or inspections of suppliers' facilities to verify compliance with quality standards, regulatory requirements, and any specific contractual obligations. This may involve assessing their infrastructure, quality control measures, personnel qualifications, and adherence to Good Manufacturing Practices (GMP) or other relevant standards.

4. **Documentation and Recordkeeping:** Maintain detailed documentation of the supplier qualification process, including evaluation criteria, assessment results, audit reports, and any corrective actions taken. These records serve as evidence of due diligence in supplier selection.

5. **Supplier Agreements and Contracts:** Establish clear and comprehensive agreements or contracts with qualified suppliers that outline expectations, quality requirements, delivery terms, pricing, dispute resolution mechanisms, and any other relevant terms and conditions.

Supplier Control:

Once suppliers are qualified, it is crucial to implement effective controls to ensure ongoing compliance with quality standards and regulatory requirements. Supplier control activities include:

1. **Supplier Performance Monitoring:** Continuously monitor the performance of suppliers to ensure they consistently meet quality standards and delivery expectations. This may involve regular performance reviews, scorecards, or Key Performance Indicators (KPIs) to measure and track supplier performance over time.

2. **Supplier Audits and Assessments:** Conduct periodic audits or assessments of suppliers to verify their continued compliance with quality standards, regulatory requirements, and contractual obligations. These audits may include assessing quality control processes, manufacturing practices, and documentation systems.

3. **Corrective Actions and Continuous Improvement:** Address any identified non-conformities or performance issues through appropriate corrective actions. Collaborate with suppliers to implement corrective measures and monitor their effectiveness. Encourage ongoing improvement by sharing best practices, providing feedback, and fostering a culture of continuous improvement.

4. **Change Control Management:** Establish robust change control procedures to manage any changes introduced by suppliers, such as changes in manufacturing processes, materials, or personnel. Evaluate the impact of supplier-initiated changes on product quality and regulatory compliance, and ensure proper documentation, evaluation, and approval of such changes.

5. **Supplier Communication and Collaboration:** Maintain open and effective communication channels with suppliers to foster collaboration, address concerns, and ensure alignment regarding quality requirements and expectations. Regularly communicate any updates, changes, or new regulatory requirements that may impact suppliers' obligations.

6. **Supplier Risk Management:** Assess and manage the risks associated with suppliers, considering factors such as their criticality, geographical location, business continuity plans, and potential impact on product quality and patient safety. Implement risk mitigation strategies and contingency plans as necessary.

By implementing robust supplier qualification and control processes, healthcare organizations can ensure a reliable supply chain, mitigate risks associated with external suppliers, and maintain consistent product quality and patient safety. Regular monitoring, evaluation, and collaboration with suppliers are essential to fostering a mutually beneficial and quality-focused relationship.

Chapter 06

Continuous Improvement and Lessons Learned

Continuous improvement is a fundamental principle of risk-based quality management in healthcare. It involves the ongoing evaluation, monitoring, and enhancement of processes, systems, and practices to drive improvements in quality, efficiency, and patient outcomes. This chapter explores the importance of continuous improvement and highlights the value of learning from past experiences through a structured approach to lessons learned.

Establishing A Culture Of Continuous Improvement

Establishing a culture of continuous improvement is vital for organizations in the healthcare industry to foster a mindset of innovation, learning, and growth. Here are some key elements and strategies for creating such a culture (Figure 6.1):

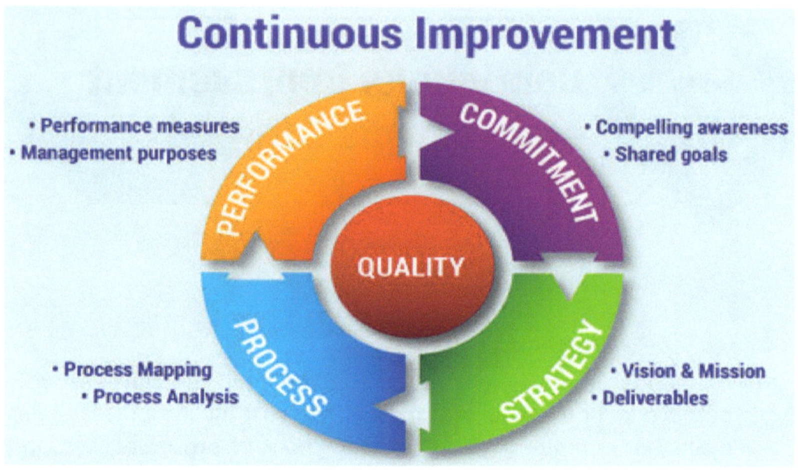

▲ **Figure 6.1**: Establishing Continuous Improvement

1. **Leadership Commitment:** Leaders must demonstrate a strong commitment to continuous improvement by actively supporting and participating in improvement initiatives. They should communicate the importance of continuous improvement, set clear expectations, and allocate resources to support improvement efforts.

2. **Employee Engagement:** Engage employees at all levels of the organization by involving them in improvement initiatives and decision-making processes. Encourage their active participation, provide opportunities for input and feedback, and recognize and celebrate their contributions. This engagement fosters a sense of ownership and accountability for driving improvements. (Table 6.1)

3. **Open Communication:** Establish open and transparent communication channels that encourage employees to share their ideas, suggestions, and concerns. Create forums for dialogue, such as regular team meetings, suggestion boxes, or online platforms, where employees can share their insights and contribute to improvement discussions.

4. **Continuous Training and Development:** Provide regular training and development opportunities to enhance employees' skills and knowledge in areas related to continuous improvement. Offer workshops, seminars, or online courses on quality improvement methodologies, problem-solving techniques, data analysis, and

other relevant topics. This empowers employees to participate in improvement projects actively and equips them with the tools needed to drive change.

5. **Learning from Failure:** Foster a culture that views failure as an opportunity for learning and growth rather than punishment. Encourage employees to share their experiences and lessons learned from unsuccessful initiatives, emphasizing the importance of analyzing failures to identify causes and prevent recurrence. Celebrate both successes and lessons learned, highlighting the value of continuous learning and improvement.

6. **Data-Driven Decision-Making:** Promote the use of data and evidence in decision-making processes. Encourage employees to collect, analyze, and interpret data to identify improvement opportunities, measure the impact of changes, and track progress over time. Provide training on data analysis techniques and make data easily accessible to support evidence-based decision-making.

7. **Recognition and Rewards:** Recognize and reward individuals and teams who actively contribute to continuous improvement efforts. Acknowledge their achievements and publicly celebrate successful improvement initiatives. This recognition can take the form of monetary rewards, certificates, or public appreciation, reinforcing the importance of continuous improvement within the organization.

8. **Continuous Improvement Frameworks:** Implement structured frameworks, such as Plan-Do-Check-Act (PDCA) or Define-Measure-Analyze-Improve-Control (DMAIC), to guide improvement initiatives. These frameworks provide a systematic approach to problem-solving, ensuring that improvement efforts are focused, measurable, and sustainable. (Table 6.3)

9. **Collaboration and Cross-Functional Teams:** Encourage collaboration and teamwork across departments and disciplines. Establish cross-functional improvement teams that bring together individuals with diverse expertise to tackle complex problems. This promotes knowledge sharing, fosters creativity, and generates innovative solutions.

10. **Continuous Improvement Metrics:** Establish key performance indicators (KPIs) and metrics that align with the organization's strategic goals and continuous improvement objectives. Regularly track and report on these metrics to assess progress, identify areas for further improvement, and communicate the impact of improvement initiatives to stakeholders. (Table 6.2)

By implementing these strategies, healthcare organizations can create a culture that values continuous improvement, embraces change, and continuously seeks opportunities to enhance quality, efficiency, and patient outcomes. A strong culture of continuous improvement empowers employees, enhances organizational performance, and drives sustainable success in the dynamic healthcare landscape.

▼ **Table 6.1**: Examples of Employee Engagement Initiatives

Initiative	Description
Improvement suggestion program	Establish a formal system for employees to submit improvement ideas and suggestions. Provide recognition and rewards for implemented suggestions.
Cross-functional improvement teams	Create cross-functional teams that bring together employees from different departments to work on improvement projects. Encourage collaboration and diverse perspectives.
Continuous improvement training	Offer regular training sessions on continuous improvement methodologies, problem-solving techniques, and data analysis. Empower employees with the skills needed to drive improvement.
Employee recognition program	Implement a program to recognize and reward employees who actively contribute to continuous improvement initiatives. Celebrate their achievements and communicate their impact.

▼ **Table 6.2**: Key Performance Indicators (kpis) for Continuous Improvement

KPI	Description
Number of improvement projects initiated	Measure the number of improvement projects initiated by employees or teams. Monitor the quantity and diversity of improvement initiatives across the organization.
Cost savings from improvement initiatives	Track the financial impact of improvement projects by measuring cost savings or cost avoidance resulting from process improvements or waste reduction.
Employee engagement survey results	Conduct regular employee engagement surveys to measure employees' perception of the organization's commitment to continuous improvement and their level of involvement in improvement initiatives.
Implementation success rate	Measure the percentage of improvement projects successfully implemented and sustained over time. Assess the organization's ability to turn ideas into tangible improvements.

▼ **Table 6.3**: Examples of Continuous Improvement Communication Channels

Communication Channel	Description
Improvement suggestion box	Provide physical or digital suggestion boxes where employees can anonymously submit improvement ideas and suggestions. Ensure a process for reviewing and responding to submissions.
Continuous improvement newsletter	Distribute a regular newsletter highlighting improvement initiatives, success stories, and upcoming opportunities for employees to get involved.
Team huddles and meetings	Incorporate dedicated time during team huddles or department meetings to discuss improvement initiatives, share updates, and address any challenges or barriers.
Online collaboration platforms	Implement an online platform where employees can share ideas, collaborate on improvement projects, and provide feedback on ongoing initiatives.

These tables provide examples of different elements related to establishing a culture of continuous improvement.

Feedback Loops And Risk Reviews

Feedback loops and risk reviews are crucial components of a robust risk-based quality management system. They help organizations continuously monitor and evaluate the effectiveness of their risk mitigation strategies and identify opportunities for improvement. Here's an overview of feedback loops and risk reviews:

1. **Feedback Loops:**

   Feedback loops are mechanisms that enable organizations to gather feedback from various sources and stakeholders, including employees, customers, regulatory agencies, and other relevant parties. These feedback loops provide valuable insights into the effectiveness of risk mitigation measures and help identify potential areas of concern or improvement. Here are some examples of feedback loops:

   - **Employee Feedback:** Establish channels for employees to provide feedback on risk management processes, procedures, and their implementation. This can include regular employee surveys, suggestion boxes, or open-door policies that encourage employees to share their observations and suggestions. (Table 6.4)

- **Customer Feedback:** Collect feedback from customers and patients regarding their experiences and perceptions of risk management in healthcare settings. This can be done through patient satisfaction surveys, feedback forms, or patient focus groups, allowing organizations to identify any gaps in risk mitigation practices from the patient's perspective. (Table 6.5)

- **Incident Reporting Systems:** Implement robust incident reporting systems that allow employees to report any incidents, near misses, or adverse events related to risk management. These systems enable the organization to capture and analyze data on incidents, identify patterns or trends, and take corrective actions to prevent recurrences.

- **External Stakeholder Feedback:** Engage with external stakeholders, such as regulatory agencies, industry associations, and accrediting bodies, to obtain feedback on risk management practices. This can involve participating in audits, inspections, or certification processes, and actively seeking input and recommendations for improvement.

2. **Risk Reviews:**

Risk reviews involve systematic and periodic assessments of risks to ensure that risk management strategies and controls remain effective. These reviews help organizations identify emerging risks, evaluate the performance of existing controls, and determine the need for additional or modified risk mitigation measures. Here are key considerations for conducting risk reviews (Table 6.6):

- **Regular Review Schedule:** Establish a predefined schedule for conducting risk reviews, considering factors such as the complexity of the healthcare environment, the nature of risks involved, and regulatory requirements. This ensures that risk reviews are conducted consistently and promptly.

- **Risk Identification:** Identify and assess new or emerging risks that may impact the organization's objectives, compliance requirements, or patient safety. This can involve reviewing incident reports, analyzing near misses, conducting risk assessments, and staying updated on industry trends and best practices.

- **Control Evaluation:** Evaluate the effectiveness of existing risk controls and mitigation measures. This may include reviewing standard operating procedures, conducting audits or inspections, analyzing data on control performance, and seeking feedback from relevant stakeholders.

- **Risk Mitigation Updates:** Based on the findings of risk reviews, update risk mitigation strategies and controls as necessary. This may involve revising policies and procedures, enhancing staff training programs, implementing new technologies or best practices, or reallocating resources to address identified gaps.

- **Documentation and Reporting:** Document the findings of risk reviews, including identified risks, control evaluations, and action plans for improvement. Report the outcomes of risk reviews to relevant stakeholders, such as management, quality committees, and regulatory agencies, as required.

By incorporating feedback loops and conducting regular risk reviews, healthcare organizations can continuously improve their risk-based quality management practices, enhance patient safety, and ensure compliance with regulatory requirements. These processes contribute to a culture of learning, adaptation, and continuous improvement within the organization.

▼ **Table 6.4**: Employee Feedback Channels

Feedback Channel	Description
Employee Surveys	Conduct regular surveys to gather feedback on risk management processes, procedures, and implementation.
Suggestion Box	Provide a physical or digital suggestion box where employees can anonymously submit suggestions and observations related to risk management.
Open-door Policy	Encourage employees to share their feedback and concerns directly with management or designated risk management personnel.

▼ **Table 6.5**: Customer Feedback Channels

Feedback Channel	Description
Patient Satisfaction Surveys	Administer surveys to gather feedback from patients regarding their experiences and perceptions of risk management in healthcare settings.
Feedback Forms	Provide feedback forms to patients, allowing them to provide input and suggestions on risk management practices.
Patient Focus Groups	Organize focus groups with a diverse range of patients to gain deeper insights into their perceptions and expectations related to risk management.

These tables provide a structured format for presenting information related to feedback channels.

Utilizing Data-driven Insights For Risk Management Enhancements

Utilizing data-driven insights is crucial for enhancing risk management practices in healthcare. By analyzing and interpreting data, organizations can identify patterns, trends, and potential areas of improvement, leading to more effective risk mitigation strategies. Here are some key aspects of utilizing data-driven insights for risk management enhancements:

1. **Data Collection and Management:**

    Establish robust systems and processes for collecting and managing relevant data. This may include incident reporting systems, quality management databases, electronic health records, and other sources of data within the organization. Ensure data integrity, accuracy, and confidentiality to maintain the reliability of the insights derived from the data.

2. **Key Risk Indicators (KRIs):**

    Define and track Key Risk Indicators specific to the organization's risk profile. These KRIs should be measurable, objective, and aligned with the organization's goals and regulatory requirements. Examples of KRIs include the frequency and severity of incidents, compliance deviations, patient complaints, and other relevant metrics. Regularly monitor and analyze these KRIs to identify areas that require attention or improvement (Table 6.6).

3. **Data Analysis Techniques:**

   Utilize various data analysis techniques to gain insights and identify patterns. Some common techniques include statistical analysis, trend analysis, root cause analysis, and data visualization. These techniques help in identifying correlations, potential causes of risks, and areas where risk mitigation strategies can be enhanced (Table 6.7).

4. **Risk Prediction and Forecasting:**

   Leverage historical data and predictive analytics to forecast potential risks and their likelihood. By analyzing past incidents, near-misses, and other relevant data, organizations can identify trends and patterns that may indicate future risks. This allows for proactive risk management by implementing preventive measures and targeted interventions.

5. **Bench-marking and Comparative Analysis:**

   Compare risk management performance with industry benchmarks and best practices. This helps organizations understand their relative position and identify areas for improvement. Comparative analysis can be done by reviewing published industry reports, participating in bench-marking initiatives, or collaborating with peers to exchange insights and lessons learned.

6. **Data-Driven Decision-Making:**

   Utilize data-driven insights to make informed decisions regarding risk management enhancements. By analyzing the data, organizations can identify high-priority risks, allocate resources effectively, and prioritize improvement initiatives based on their potential impact. Data-driven decision-making ensures that risk management efforts are targeted and aligned with the organization's overall objectives.

7. **Continuous Monitoring and Review:**

   Continuously monitor and review the effectiveness of risk management enhancements based on data-driven insights. Regularly reassess and update risk mitigation strategies as new data becomes available. This iterative process allows for ongoing improvement and ensures that risk management practices remain aligned with changing organizational needs and evolving industry standards.

By harnessing the power of data-driven insights, healthcare organizations can enhance their risk management practices, improve patient safety, and drive continuous improvement. The systematic analysis of data enables organizations to identify risks proactively, implement targeted interventions, and continuously refine their risk management strategies.

▼ **Table 6.6**: Key Risk Indicators (KRIS)

KRI	Description
Number of Incidents	Track the frequency of incidents and near misses to identify trends and areas requiring improved risk mitigation.
Compliance Deviations	Monitor deviations from regulatory requirements or internal policies to identify potential compliance risks and areas for improvement.
Patient Complaints	Track patient complaints related to safety incidents, adverse events, or other risk-related issues to identify areas for improvement.
Trend Analysis	Analyze historical data to identify trends and patterns in risk events, allowing proactive risk management and preventive measures.
Employee Training Completion	Monitor the completion rates of employee training programs on risk management to ensure compliance and assess the effectiveness of training efforts.

▼ **Table 6.7**: Data Analysis Techniques

Data Analysis Technique	Description
Statistical Analysis	Utilize statistical methods to identify correlations, distributions, and trends within risk-related data sets.
Root Cause Analysis	Conduct in-depth analysis of incidents or adverse events to identify underlying causes and contributing factors.
Data Visualization	Use visual tools such as charts, graphs, and dashboards to represent risk-related data in a clear and understandable manner.
Predictive Analytics	Apply advanced analytics techniques to forecast potential risks and their likelihood based on historical data and patterns.
Comparative Analysis	Compare risk management performance and outcomes against industry benchmarks and best practices to identify areas for improvement.

These tables provide a structured format for presenting information related to key risk indicators and data analysis techniques.

Incorporating Lessons Learned Into Risk Management Practices

Incorporating lessons learned into risk management practices is essential for continuous improvement and proactive risk mitigation. Lessons learned from past incidents, near misses, audits, and other experiences provide valuable insights that can help organizations identify weaknesses, enhance existing controls, and prevent similar risks in the future. Here are key steps to incorporate lessons learned into risk management practices:

1. **Documentation of Lessons Learned:**

   Establish a systematic process for documenting and capturing lessons learned from various sources, such as incident reports, root cause analyses, post-market surveillance, and internal or external audits. Ensure that these lessons learned are well-documented and easily accessible to relevant stakeholders involved in risk management (Table 6.8).

2. **Knowledge Sharing and Communication:**

   Facilitate knowledge sharing and communication channels within the organization to disseminate lessons learned effectively. This can include conducting regular risk management meetings, sharing reports and case studies, organizing workshops or training sessions, and utilizing collaboration tools to encourage open discussions and information exchange.

3. **Risk Register Updates:**

   Regularly review and update the risk register or risk database to incorporate new risks identified through lessons learned. Assess the impact of these risks and assign appropriate risk levels. Link the lessons learned to specific risks, enabling easy reference and tracking of actions taken to address those risks.

4. **Root Cause Analysis and Corrective Actions:**

   Perform thorough root cause analyses for incidents or near misses and identify underlying causes and contributing factors. Based on the findings, develop and implement appropriate corrective actions to address the causes and prevent recurrence. Document these actions and track their implementation and effectiveness.

5. **Training and Education:**

   Utilize lessons learned to enhance training and education programs related to risk management. Incorporate real-life examples, case studies, and lessons learned into training materials and sessions. This helps to increase awareness, knowledge, and competency among staff members, enabling them to identify better and manage risks in their day-to-day activities.

6. **Process and Procedure Improvements:**

   Review existing risk management processes and procedures in light of lessons learned. Identify areas where process improvements or procedural changes can be made to strengthen risk mitigation efforts. Incorporate lessons learned into these updates and ensure that revised processes are communicated and implemented across the organization (Table 6.9).

7. **Continuous Monitoring and Evaluation:**

   Continuously monitor the effectiveness of lessons learned in improving risk management practices. Regularly evaluate the impact of the implemented corrective actions and process improvements. Adjust and refine risk management strategies based on ongoing evaluation, incorporating new lessons learned as they arise.

8. **Feedback and Continuous Improvement Loop:**

   Establish a feedback loop to gather input from stakeholders regarding the effectiveness of lessons learned and their impact on risk management. Encourage staff members to provide feedback, share their experiences, and suggest further improvements. Actively seek opportunities for continuous improvement based on this feedback.

By incorporating lessons learned into risk management practices, organizations can proactively identify and mitigate risks, prevent future incidents, and foster a culture of continuous learning and improvement. Lessons learned serve as valuable inputs for refining risk management strategies, strengthening controls, and ultimately enhancing patient safety and quality of care.

▼ **Table 6.8**: Lessons Learned Documentation

Incident/ Near Miss	Lesson Learned	Action Taken	Root Cause Analysis	Corrective Actions
Example Incident 1	Improved communication among team members to prevent miscommunication.	Implemented regular team huddles and standardized handover procedures.	Misinterpretation of medication orders due to illegible handwriting.	Implemented electronic prescribing system and mandatory handwriting legibility guidelines.
Example Incident 2	Lack of clear accountability for risk mitigation measures.	Updated roles and responsibilities, and established clear accountability framework.	Failure to follow established procedures during equipment sterilization.	Conducted retraining on equipment sterilization procedures and implemented improved documentation and verification processes.
Example Near Miss	Inadequate equipment maintenance contributed to potential safety risks.	Revised maintenance schedule and implemented proactive equipment inspections.	Inadequate staff training on handling hazardous substances.	Enhanced staff training programs on proper handling, storage, and disposal of hazardous substances.

▼ **Table 6.9**: Process and Procedure Improvements

Process/Procedure	Lessons Learned	Improvements Implemented
Incident Reporting	Inconsistent reporting and follow-up processes.	Streamlined incident reporting procedures and implemented standardized follow-up protocols.
Risk Assessment	Lack of comprehensive risk assessment documentation.	Updated risk assessment templates and provided clear guidance on documentation requirements.
Communication Channels	Insufficient communication channels for sharing lessons learned.	Established a centralized platform for sharing lessons learned and best practices.

These tables provide a structured format for presenting information related to lessons learned, root cause analysis, and process improvements.

Case Studies and Practical Examples

In this chapter, we will explore a series of case studies and practical examples that highlight the application of risk-based quality management principles in the healthcare industry. These real-world scenarios provide valuable insights into the challenges faced by healthcare professionals and the strategies employed to effectively manage risks while maintaining quality and regulatory compliance. By examining these case studies, readers will gain a deeper understanding of how risk-based quality management principles can be implemented in different healthcare settings.

Real-world Case Studies Highlighting Successful Risk-based Quality Management Implementations

Case Study 1: Implementation of Risk Management in a Hospital Setting

Background:

A large urban hospital recognized the need to enhance patient safety and improve overall quality of care through the implementation of a risk-based quality management system. The hospital faced challenges related to patient falls, medication errors, and healthcare-associated infections. They embarked on a comprehensive risk management initiative to address these issues. (Table 7.1)

Implementation Strategy:

1. **Risk Identification:** The hospital conducted a thorough assessment of potential risks across various departments and clinical processes. This involved engaging frontline staff, conducting incident reporting and analysis, and leveraging data from patient safety indicators.

2. **Risk Assessment:** Identified risks were assessed using a systematic approach, taking into consideration severity, probability, and detectability. The hospital utilized tools such as Failure Mode and Effects Analysis (FMEA) and Hazard Analysis and Critical Control Points (HACCP) to assess risks and prioritize mitigation efforts.

3. **Risk Mitigation Strategies:** The hospital implemented targeted risk mitigation strategies based on the identified risks. This included staff education and training programs, improved communication protocols, standardization of procedures, implementation of safety checklists, and the use of technology solutions to reduce medication errors.

4. **Integration with Quality Management Systems:** Risk management was integrated into existing quality management systems to ensure a coordinated and comprehensive approach. Risk management became an integral part of performance improvement initiatives, clinical guidelines, and incident management processes.

Results and Benefits:

- Significant reduction in patient falls and medication errors due to targeted risk mitigation efforts.

- Decreased rates of healthcare-associated infections through improved infection prevention protocols and surveillance systems.

- Enhanced communication and teamwork among staff, leading to improved patient outcomes and increased patient satisfaction.

- Regulatory compliance and accreditation success due to the establishment of robust risk management processes and documentation.

Lessons Learned:

- Engaging frontline staff and involving them in risk identification and mitigation processes is crucial for successful implementation.

- Integration of risk management into existing quality management systems enhances effectiveness and ensures a holistic approach.

- Continuous monitoring and evaluation of risk management processes allow for ongoing improvement and adaptation.

▼ **Table 7.1**: Case Study 1 - Implementation of Risk Management in a Hospital Setting

Risk Area	Identified Risks	Mitigation Strategies	Results/Benefits
Patient Falls	Slippery floors, inadequate lighting	Installation of non-slip flooring, improved lighting, implementation of fall prevention protocols	50% reduction in patient falls in the first year
Medication Errors	Illegible handwriting, lack of double-check procedures	Electronic prescribing system, mandatory double-checks for high-risk medications	30% reduction in medication errors
Healthcare-associated Infections	Inadequate hand hygiene, improper disinfection protocols	Staff education on hand hygiene, implementation of standardized disinfection protocols	25% decrease in healthcare-associated infections

Case Study 2: Compliance with ISO 13485 and EU MDR for a Medical Device Manufacturer

Background:

A medical device manufacturing company aimed to achieve compliance with ISO 13485 and the European Medical Device Regulation (EU MDR). The company recognized the importance of risk-based approaches in product development, manufacturing, and post-market surveillance. (Table 7.2)

Implementation Strategy:

1. **Gap Analysis:** The company conducted a comprehensive gap analysis to identify areas of non-compliance with ISO 13485 and EU MDR. This included assessing the existing quality management system, documentation, and processes against the regulatory requirements.

2. **Risk-Based Product Development:** The company implemented risk management activities throughout the product development lifecycle, including risk assessment, risk control strategies, and risk evaluation. This involved utilizing tools such as FMEA, risk matrices, and risk management plans.

3. **Supplier Qualification and Control:** The company established rigorous supplier qualification processes to ensure that suppliers met the required quality and regulatory standards. Risk assessments were conducted for critical suppliers, and ongoing supplier performance monitoring was implemented.

4. **Post-Market Surveillance:** The company implemented a robust post-market surveillance system to monitor the performance and safety of its devices in the market. This involved the collection and analysis of data from adverse event reporting, customer complaints, and other feedback channels.

Results and Benefits:

- Successful achievement of ISO 13485 and EU MDR compliance, ensuring access to European markets and maintaining customer confidence.

- Enhanced product safety through the implementation of risk-based product development and post-market surveillance processes.

- Improved supplier management and control, leading to a more reliable supply chain and reduced risks associated with supplier quality.

S. No	Hazard	Hazardous situation	Severity Level	Possibility of Occurrence	Risk	Risk Evaluation/Acceptability Decision	Risk Control Option	Implementation of Risk Control	Residual Risk Severity	Occurrence after Risk	Residual Risk Acceptance	Risk acceptance after risk control measure	Information supplied to user/patient	Risk arising from risk control measure
1a	Dimensional variations in predicate and subject device	Inadequate Measurement Improper dimensional input	S4	O3	Not Acceptable	Dimensional variation with predicate device is not acceptable as it may lead to device failure or revision surgery	Design review Drawing is to be control and approval before transfer to production	Design review Procedure for Design Review A3-DND-QP-xxx Controlling & Approval of drawing covered under A3-DND-QP-xxx Procedure for 3D, 2D Model & Drawing preparation.	S4	O1	ALAP	With strict compliance with Design and Development controlling all D&D stages: input, output, review, verification, validation and design transfer, current risk is acceptable	Not Applicable	No

▲ **Figure 7.1**: Utilization of Fmea Tool

Lessons Learned:

- Thorough gap analysis is essential to identify areas of non-compliance and develop targeted strategies for compliance.

- Risk-based approaches should be integrated into all stages of product development and post-market surveillance for effective risk management.

- Establishing strong supplier qualification and control processes is critical for ensuring the quality and safety of medical devices.

These case studies demonstrate the successful implementation of risk-based quality management principles in healthcare settings, leading to improved patient safety, enhanced quality of care, and regulatory compliance. They highlight the importance of risk identification, assessment, and mitigation, as well as the integration of risk management into existing quality management systems. By learning from these real-world examples, healthcare professionals can gain insights and inspiration to implement effective risk-based quality management practices in their own organizations.

▼ **Table 7.2**: Case Study 2 - Compliance with ISO 13485 and EU MDR for a Medical Device Manufacturer

Compliance Area	Gap Analysis Findings	Corrective Actions Implemented	Results/Benefits
Quality Management System	Incomplete documentation, lack of risk-based approaches	Updated quality management system documentation, implemented risk management procedures	Achieved ISO 13485 and EU MDR compliance
Risk-Based Product Development	Insufficient risk assessment and control strategies	Implemented risk assessment tools, integrated risk management into product development processes	Enhanced product safety and regulatory compliance
Supplier Qualification and Control	Inconsistent supplier qualification processes	Implemented rigorous supplier qualification procedures, ongoing performance monitoring	Improved supplier quality and reliability

Lessons Learned And Best Practices From Healthcare Organizations

Lessons learned and best practices from healthcare organizations play a crucial role in improving risk-based quality management. Here are some examples. (Table 7.3 and 7.4)

1. **Engage Frontline Staff:**

   - Best Practice: Actively involve frontline staff in the risk identification and mitigation processes. They have valuable insights and firsthand knowledge of potential risks in their areas of work.

   - Example: Conduct regular safety huddles or risk assessment meetings where staff can openly discuss and report potential risks, contributing to a culture of safety.

2. **Integration of Risk Management:**

- Best Practice: Integrate risk management into existing quality management systems and processes to ensure a holistic approach.

- Example: Establish clear linkages between risk management and other quality improvement initiatives, such as incident reporting, root cause analysis, and performance improvement projects.

3. **Data-Driven Decision-Making:**

- Best Practice: Utilize data and analytics to identify trends, patterns, and areas of improvement for risk management.

- Example: Implement a robust data collection and analysis system to track and monitor risk indicators, adverse events, and near misses, enabling proactive risk mitigation strategies.

4. **Collaboration and Communication:**

- Best Practice: Foster a culture of collaboration and open communication across all levels of the organization to enhance risk management effectiveness.

- Example: Establish multidisciplinary risk management teams or committees that include representatives from various departments and stakeholders, facilitating effective communication and collaboration.

5. **Continuous Training and Education:**

- Best Practice: Provide ongoing training and education to staff on risk management principles, tools, and techniques.

- Example: Conduct regular training sessions, workshops, and webinars to keep staff updated on risk assessment methods, incident reporting protocols, and the importance of proactive risk mitigation.

6. Monitoring and Evaluation:

- **Best Practice:** Implement a robust monitoring and evaluation process to assess the effectiveness of risk management strategies and identify areas for improvement.

- **Example:** Conduct regular audits, internal reviews, and performance evaluations to assess compliance with risk management protocols and identify opportunities for enhancement.

7. Regulatory Compliance:

- **Best Practice:** Stay updated with regulatory requirements and standards relevant to the healthcare industry.

- **Example:** Assign a dedicated team or individual responsible for monitoring and interpreting changes in regulations, ensuring timely compliance with ISO standards, EU MDR, FDA guidelines, or other relevant regulatory frameworks.

By including these lessons learned and best practices in the book, healthcare professionals can gain valuable insights and practical guidance for implementing risk-based quality management effectively in their organizations.

▼ **Table 7.3**: Best Practices for Effective Risk Mitigation

Risk Mitigation Best Practice	Description
Standardization of Procedures	Establish standardized processes and protocols to reduce variation and potential risks
Robust Incident Reporting and Analysis	Implement a system for reporting and analyzing incidents to identify root causes and implement corrective actions
Ongoing Staff Education and Training	Provide regular training on risk management principles and safe practices
Effective Communication and Teamwork	Foster a culture of open communication and collaboration to enhance risk identification and resolution

Risk Mitigation Best Practice	Description
Continuous Monitoring and Auditing	Implement regular monitoring and auditing processes to ensure compliance and identify areas for improvement
Proactive Equipment Maintenance and Inspections	Develop a preventive maintenance schedule and conduct regular equipment inspections to mitigate equipment-related risks
Implementing Technology Solutions	Utilize technology solutions to automate processes, enhance data analysis, and improve risk monitoring
Patient and Family Engagement	Involve patients and their families in the care process, encourage feedback, and integrate patient preferences into risk management strategies.

This table provides a concise and organized overview of the best practices for effective Risk Mitigation. They serve as quick references for healthcare professionals, enabling them to identify and implement effective strategies for risk mitigation in their respective organizations.

Analyzing Challenges And Solutions In Different Healthcare Contexts

Analyzing challenges and identifying solutions in different healthcare contexts is crucial for effective risk-based quality management. Here are some examples of challenges and potential solutions.

Challenge 1: Resource Constraints

- Context: Healthcare organizations operating in resource-constrained settings face challenges in allocating sufficient resources for risk management activities.

- Solution: Prioritize and allocate resources based on risk assessment outcomes. Focus on high-risk areas and develop targeted strategies for risk mitigation. Seek partnerships and collaborations with external organizations to leverage additional resources and expertise.

Challenge 2: Diverse Stakeholders

- Context: Healthcare environments involve multiple stakeholders with different priorities and perspectives, such as healthcare providers, patients, regulatory bodies, and insurance companies.

- Solution: Foster effective communication and collaboration among stakeholders. Establish clear lines of communication and channels for feedback. Encourage shared decision-making and involvement of stakeholders in risk management processes to ensure a comprehensive and inclusive approach.

Challenge 3: Technology Integration

- Context: Incorporating new technologies and digital solutions into existing healthcare systems can pose challenges in terms of data security, interoperability, and staff training.

- Solution: Develop a robust technology integration strategy that includes thorough risk assessments, data privacy protocols, and training programs for staff. Ensure interoperability of systems and establish effective data governance frameworks to mitigate potential risks associated with technology implementation.

Challenge 4: Regulatory Compliance

- Context: Keeping up with evolving regulations and maintaining compliance with various standards and guidelines can be challenging for healthcare organizations.

- Solution: Establish a dedicated team or assign specific personnel responsible for monitoring regulatory changes and ensuring compliance. Conduct regular audits and internal reviews to identify gaps and implement corrective actions. Develop strong documentation and recordkeeping practices to demonstrate compliance.

Challenge 5: Cultural and Organizational Resistance

- Context: Resistance to change and lack of a culture of quality and safety can impede the adoption of risk-based quality management practices.

- Solution: Implement change management strategies to address cultural resistance. Engage and educate staff at all levels about the benefits of risk-based quality management. Foster a culture of continuous improvement and learning, where risk identification and mitigation are embraced as essential components of patient safety and quality of care.

By examining challenges and presenting potential solutions within different healthcare contexts, this book can provide valuable insights and practical guidance to healthcare professionals, enabling them to navigate the specific challenges they may encounter and implement effective risk-based quality management strategies in their respective settings.

Chapter 08

Tools and Templates

In this chapter, we will provide a comprehensive collection of tools and templates to support healthcare professionals in implementing risk-based quality management in their organizations. These tools and templates are designed to streamline and standardize risk management processes, facilitate documentation and recordkeeping, and enhance overall compliance with regulatory requirements. By utilizing these resources, healthcare professionals can save time and effort while ensuring the effectiveness and efficiency of their risk management practices.

Customizing And Applying The Provided Resources To Specific Healthcare Organizations

Customizing and applying the provided resources to specific healthcare organizations is essential to ensure their effectiveness and relevance. Here are some guidelines on how to tailor and apply the tools, templates, and checklists for risk-based quality management (Table 8.1 to 8.4):

1. **Assess Organizational Needs:** Before implementing any resource, assess the specific needs, goals, and regulatory requirements of the healthcare organization. Consider factors such as size, specialization, geographical location, and applicable regulations (e.g., ISO 13485, EU MDR) to determine which resources will be most beneficial.

2. **Customize Templates and Checklists:** Adapt the provided templates and checklists to align with the organization's terminology, processes, and unique requirements. Modify the sections, fields, or questions to capture the relevant information specific to the organization's risk management practices.

3. **Incorporate Organizational Policies and Procedures:** Integrate the resources with existing organizational policies and procedures. Ensure that the templates and checklists reflect the organization's quality management system and adhere to its internal guidelines and processes.

4. **Seek Input from Stakeholders:** Involve key stakeholders, including risk managers, quality assurance professionals, healthcare providers, and relevant staff members, in customizing and applying the resources. Their input will ensure that the tools and templates address the specific needs and challenges of the organization.

5. **Provide Clear Instructions and Guidelines:** Accompany the resources with clear instructions and guidelines on how to use them effectively. Explain the purpose, intended outcomes, and step-by-step instructions for completing the templates or using the checklists. This will help users understand how to apply the resources in their daily practices.

6. **Train and Support Users:** Offer training sessions or workshops to familiarize staff members with the customized resources. Provide guidance and ongoing support to ensure that users understand how to use the tools effectively, templates, and checklists for risk-based quality management.

7. **Regularly Review and Update:** Continuously review and update the resources based on feedback, lessons learned, and changes in regulations or organizational needs. Stay informed about industry best practices and evolving standards to ensure the resources remain relevant and effective.

By customizing and applying the provided resources to specific healthcare organizations, you can enhance their value and maximize their impact on risk-based quality management practices. Remember that these resources should serve as a starting point, and it's crucial to adapt them to fit the unique requirements and context of each organization.

▼ **Table 8.1**: Customization Guidelines for Templates and Checklists

Resource	Customization Guidelines
Risk Assessment Matrix	Adapt the severity and probability rating scales to align with the organization's risk assessment approach.
Risk Management Plan	Customize the objectives, strategies, and action plans to reflect the organization's specific goals
Incident Reporting Form	Modify the fields and categories to capture organization-specific information during incident reporting
Internal Audit Checklist	Tailor the checklist questions to match the organization's regulatory requirements and internal policies

▼ **Table 8.2**: Stakeholder Involvement in Customization Process

Stakeholder Role	Involvement in Customization Process
Risk Managers	Provide insights on organization-specific risk management practices and required documentation
Quality Assurance Team	Review and align the templates and checklists with existing quality management processes and systems
Healthcare Providers	Offer feedback on the usability and relevance of the resources in their daily clinical workflows
Staff Members	Participate in training sessions and provide feedback on the customization of the resources

▼ **Table 8.3**: Training and Support for Resource Implementation

Training and Support Activities	Description
Resource Training Sessions	Conduct training sessions to explain the purpose, usage, and customization guidelines for each resource
User Guides and Instructions	Provide comprehensive user guides and instructions to help users navigate and utilize the resources.
Ongoing Support and Helpdesk Assistance	Offer ongoing support and a dedicated help desk to address any questions or issues related to the resources.

▼ **Table 8.4**: Review and Update Process for Resources

Review and Update Activities	Description
Feedback Collection Mechanisms	Establish feedback channels to gather input and suggestions from users regarding the effectiveness of the resources.
Periodic Review and Revision	Conduct regular reviews of the resources to ensure they remain up-to-date with changing regulations and best practices.
Version Control and Documentation	Maintain a version control system and document changes made to the resources for transparency and traceability

Documentation Examples And Guidelines For Risk Management Practices

Some examples of documentation and guidelines for risk management practices in healthcare organizations are mentioned below:

1. **Risk Management Policy:**

   - Clearly state the organization's commitment to risk management and its integration into all processes and activities.

   - Define the objectives, scope, and responsibilities related to risk management.

   - Specify the regulatory requirements and standards to which the organization adheres.

2. **Risk Management Plan:**

   - Outline the overall approach and methodology for risk management.

   - Describe the processes for risk identification, assessment, mitigation, and monitoring.

   - Define the roles and responsibilities of individuals involved in risk management.

   - Establish the criteria for risk prioritization and decision-making.

   - Detail the communication and reporting procedures for risk-related information.

3. **Risk Register:**

    - Capture and record identified risks, including their description, likelihood, severity, and current risk status.

    - Assign responsibility for each risk and track the progress of mitigation measures.

    - Include a system for regularly reviewing and updating the risk register.

4. **Risk Assessment Reports:**

    - Document the results of risk assessments, including the identified risks, their potential impacts, and the likelihood of occurrence.

    - Provide an analysis of risk severity and prioritize risks based on their significance.

    - Recommend appropriate risk mitigation measures and strategies.

5. **Incident Reporting and Investigation:**

    - Develop incident reporting forms to capture information about incidents, accidents, or near-misses.

    - Define a process for reporting incidents and conducting investigations to identify causes and contributing factors.

    - Document the findings and corrective actions taken to address identified risks and prevent recurrence.

6. **Risk Communication Plan:**

    - Specify the methods and channels for communicating risk-related information to stakeholders, including staff, patients, and regulatory authorities.

    - Define the frequency and content of risk communication, considering the sensitivity and significance of the risks.

    - Ensure that risk communication is clear, accurate, and timely to facilitate informed decision-making.

7. **Training and Awareness Materials:**

- Develop training materials and resources to educate staff on risk management principles, processes, and best practices.

- Provide guidelines and procedures for staff to follow when encountering potential risks or adverse events.

- Raise awareness about the importance of risk management and encourage a culture of reporting and learning from risks.

The documentation examples and guidelines should be tailored to the specific needs and requirements of the healthcare organization and regulatory frameworks they operate within. They should align with the organization's risk management policies and processes, as well as applicable industry standards and guidelines.

Chapter 09

Future Considerations

In the rapidly evolving healthcare landscape, it is crucial for healthcare professionals to anticipate and adapt to future changes and challenges in risk-based quality management. This chapter explores emerging trends, technologies, and regulatory developments that are likely to impact risk management practices in the healthcare industry. It also highlights the importance of continuous learning and proactive strategies to stay ahead of these changes.

Emerging Trends in Risk-Based Quality Management

1. **Data-driven Decision-Making:** With the increasing availability of healthcare data and advancements in analytics, there is a growing trend towards leveraging data-driven insights for risk management. Organizations are using advanced analytics tools and techniques to identify patterns, detect emerging risks, and make informed decisions to improve patient safety and outcomes. (Table 9.1)

2. **Predictive and Prescriptive Analytics:** In line with data-driven decision-making, predictive and prescriptive analytics are gaining prominence in risk-based quality management. These approaches use historical data and machine learning algorithms to forecast and prevent potential risks before they occur. By proactively identifying high-risk areas, healthcare organizations can implement targeted interventions and preventive measures.

3. **Proactive Risk Management:** Traditionally, risk management has been reactive, focusing on addressing incidents and adverse events after they occur. However, there is a shift towards proactive risk management, where organizations proactively identify and mitigate potential risks before they escalate into problems. This approach

involves conducting risk assessments, implementing preventive measures, and regularly monitoring and reassessing risks.

4. **Integration of Quality and Risk Management:** Quality management and risk management are closely intertwined. There is a growing recognition of the need to integrate these functions to achieve more holistic and effective risk-based quality management. By aligning quality objectives and processes with risk management strategies, organizations can optimize resources, streamline workflows, and enhance overall quality and safety.

5. **Human Factors and Human-Centered Design:** The role of human factors and human-centered design in risk-based quality management is gaining attention. Understanding how human behaviors, capabilities, and limitations contribute to risks can help design systems, processes, and technologies that mitigate these risks. Incorporating human factors principles into risk management practices can enhance usability, reduce errors, and improve patient safety.

6. **Collaboration and Communication:** Risk management is no longer viewed as solely the responsibility of a single department or individual. Collaboration and effective communication across different stakeholders, including healthcare providers, patients, regulatory bodies, and suppliers, are crucial for comprehensive risk-based quality management. Transparent and timely sharing of risk information facilitates proactive risk mitigation and enables a more coordinated approach.

7. **Continuous Learning and Improvement:** The importance of continuous learning and improvement in risk-based quality management cannot be overstated. Healthcare organizations are encouraged to establish mechanisms for capturing and sharing lessons learned from risk events, near misses, and best practices. This enables the identification of systemic issues, implementation of corrective actions, and the ongoing improvement of risk management processes.

These emerging trends highlight the evolving nature of risk-based quality management in healthcare. By embracing these trends and incorporating them into their practices, healthcare organizations can enhance their ability to identify, assess, and mitigate risks, ultimately improving patient safety, quality of care, and organizational performance.

▼ **Table 9.1**: Emerging Trends

EMERGING TREND	DESCRIPTION
DATA-DRIVEN DECISION-MAKING	
Increased availability	Growing accessibility and availability of healthcare data for risk management purposes
Advanced analytics	Utilizing sophisticated analytics tools and techniques for data analysis and risk assessment
Real-time monitoring	Implementing systems for real-time monitoring of key risk indicators
PROACTIVE RISK MANAGEMENT	
Risk assessments	Conducting comprehensive risk assessments to identify proactively and evaluate risks
Preventive measures	Implementing preventive measures and controls to mitigate potential risks
Ongoing monitoring	Continuously monitoring and reassessing risks to ensure timely intervention
INTEGRATION OF QUALITY AND RISK MANAGEMENT	
Alignment of objectives	Aligning quality objectives with risk management strategies to optimize resources
Streamlined workflows	Integrating quality and risk management processes to streamline workflows
Enhanced quality and safety	Improving overall quality and safety by integrating risk management into quality practices
HUMAN FACTORS AND HUMAN-CENTERED DESIGN	
Understanding behaviors	Incorporating knowledge of human behaviors, capabilities, and limitations into risk management
Usability improvements	Applying human-centered design principles to enhance usability and reduce errors
Improved patient safety	Designing systems, processes, and technologies that mitigate human-related risks
COLLABORATION AND COMMUNICATION	
Cross-stakeholder collaboration	Collaborating across different stakeholders for comprehensive risk management
Transparent risk communication	Facilitating transparent and timely communication of risk information

Contd...

EMERGING TREND	DESCRIPTION
Coordinated approach	Fostering a coordinated approach to risk mitigation and management among stakeholders
CONTINUOUS LEARNING AND IMPROVEMENT	
Lessons learned	Capturing and sharing lessons learned from risk events and near misses
Systemic issue identification	Identifying and addressing systemic issues to improve risk management processes
Continuous improvement	Implementing a culture of continuous learning and improvement in risk-based quality management

This table provides a snapshot of the emerging trends in risk-based quality management. The actual content and details may vary based on specific industry developments and organizational contexts. It's important to customize the tables to reflect the specific trends and their implications for the healthcare organization's risk management.

Technological Advancements And Their Impact On Risk Management

Technological advancements have significantly influenced risk management practices in various industries, including healthcare. Here are some examples of technological advancements and their impact on risk management:

1. **Artificial Intelligence (AI) and Machine Learning (ML):**

   - AI and ML algorithms can analyze large datasets and identify patterns, trends, and anomalies that may indicate potential risks.

   - These technologies enable predictive analytics, allowing organizations to anticipate and mitigate risks before they occur.

   - AI-powered tools can automate risk assessment processes, making them more efficient and accurate.(Table 9.2)

2. **Internet of Things (IoT):**

- IoT devices, such as wearable health trackers and remote monitoring systems, generate real-time patient data, which can be analyzed for risk identification and early intervention.

- IoT-enabled systems can provide alerts and notifications to healthcare providers in case of critical events or deviations from normal conditions, improving risk response.

3. **Telemedicine and Remote Healthcare:**

- Telemedicine platforms and remote healthcare technologies allow patients to receive care from their homes, reducing the risk of exposure to infectious diseases in healthcare facilities.

- However, these technologies also introduce new risks, such as data privacy and security concerns, which need to be effectively managed.

4. **Electronic Health Records (EHR) and Health Information Systems:**

- Digitalization of patient records and health information systems enhances the availability and accessibility of patient data for risk assessment and management.

- EHR systems facilitate the tracking of adverse events, near misses, and medication errors, enabling proactive risk mitigation strategies.

5. **Blockchain Technology:**

- Blockchain provides a secure and decentralized platform for storing and sharing sensitive healthcare data.

- Its tamper-resistant nature enhances data integrity, reduces fraud risks, and improves traceability, particularly in supply chain management and drug authentication.

6. **Robotics and Automation:**

- Robotic process automation (RPA) can automate repetitive and error-prone tasks, reducing the risk of human error.

- Surgical robots and assistive technologies can enhance precision and patient safety during complex medical procedures.

7. Data Security and Cybersecurity:

- As healthcare systems become increasingly digitized, protecting patient data and ensuring cybersecurity is crucial.

- Advancements in data encryption, access controls, and cybersecurity technologies are essential for mitigating the risks of data breaches and unauthorized access.

These technological advancements bring both opportunities and challenges to risk management in healthcare. It is important for organizations to assess the risks associated with adopting and implementing these technologies and develop robust risk management strategies to ensure patient safety, data privacy, and regulatory compliance.

▼ **Table 9.2**: Technological Advancements and Their Impact on Risk Management

TECHNOLOGICAL ADVANCEMENT	IMPACT ON RISK MANAGEMENT
ARTIFICIAL INTELLIGENCE AND MACHINE LEARNING	
Artificial Intelligence	AI algorithms can analyze large datasets to identify patterns and predict risks, improving risk assessment
Machine Learning	ML models can detect anomalies and deviations, enabling proactive risk mitigation
Automation	Automated processes reduce the risk of human error and streamline risk management workflows
INTERNET OF THINGS (IoT) AND REMOTE HEALTHCARE	
Internet of Things (IoT)	IoT devices provide real-time data for risk monitoring and early intervention
Remote Healthcare	Remote care technologies reduce the risk of patient exposure to infectious diseases and improve access to care
Data Privacy and Security	Protecting patient data in IoT and remote healthcare systems is crucial, requiring robust cybersecurity measures and privacy protocols
ELECTRONIC HEALTH RECORDS (EHR) AND HEALTH INFORMATION SYSTEMS	
Electronic Health Records	EHR systems improve risk assessment by centralizing patient data and enabling efficient tracking of adverse events and medication errors

TECHNOLOGICAL ADVANCEMENT	IMPACT ON RISK MANAGEMENT
Health Information Systems	Integrated health information systems facilitate risk communication and enhance patient safety through coordinated care and decision-making
BLOCKCHAIN TECHNOLOGY	
Blockchain Technology	Blockchain provides secure and transparent record-keeping, enhancing data integrity, traceability, and supply chain risk management.
Data Privacy and Security	Blockchain's decentralized nature improves data security and mitigates the risk of data breaches and unauthorized access
ROBOTICS AND AUTOMATION	
Robotics	Surgical robots and assistive technologies improve precision, reducing the risk of errors during medical procedures
Automation	Robotic process automation streamlines repetitive tasks, minimizing human error and optimizing risk management workflows
DATA SECURITY AND CYBERSECURITY	
Data Security	Advanced encryption and access control technologies protect patient data and mitigate the risk of data breaches and unauthorized access
Cybersecurity	Robust cybersecurity measures ensure the integrity and confidentiality of healthcare systems and data

This table provides a concise overview of how various technological advancements impact risk management in healthcare.

Evolving Regulatory Frameworks And Their Implications For Healthcare Professionals

Evolving regulatory frameworks in the healthcare industry have significant implications for healthcare professionals. Here are some examples of evolving regulatory frameworks and their implications (Table 9.13):

1.   **European Medical Device Regulation (EU MDR):**

   - Implementation of stricter regulations for medical devices in the European Union, aiming to enhance patient safety and device traceability.

   - Healthcare professionals need to ensure compliance with new requirements, such as increased clinical evidence and post-market surveillance obligations.

   - Implications include the need for updated documentation, enhanced risk management practices, and collaboration with notified bodies for device certification.

2.   **General Data Protection Regulation (GDPR):**

   - GDPR is a comprehensive data protection regulation in the European Union that governs the handling of personal data.

   - Healthcare professionals must ensure the privacy and security of patient data, including obtaining consent for data processing and implementing appropriate security measures.

   - Implications include the need for robust data protection policies, data breach reporting, and maintaining transparent data practices.

3.   **Health Insurance Portability and Accountability Act (HIPAA):**

   - HIPAA regulations in the United States aim to protect the privacy and security of patients' protected health information (PHI).

   - Healthcare professionals must adhere to HIPAA requirements when handling and transmitting PHI, including ensuring data encryption, access controls, and maintaining audit trails.

   - Implications include the need for HIPAA training, implementing privacy policies, and conducting regular risk assessments.

4. **Good Clinical Practice (GCP) Guidelines:**

    - GCP guidelines provide standards for conducting clinical trials to ensure participant safety, data integrity, and ethical practices.

    - Healthcare professionals involved in clinical research must follow GCP guidelines, including informed consent, protocol adherence, and proper documentation.

    - Implications include the need for GCP training, maintaining trial documentation, and adherence to ethical principles throughout the research process.

5. **International Organization for Standardization (ISO) Standards:**

    - ISO standards, such as ISO 9001 (Quality Management) and ISO 13485 (Medical Devices), provide frameworks for quality management systems in healthcare.

    - Healthcare professionals may need to comply with ISO standards to ensure consistent quality, risk management, and regulatory compliance.

    - Implications include the need for process documentation, risk assessment and mitigation, and continuous improvement practices.

6. **Pharmacovigilance and Drug Safety Regulations:**

    - Pharmacovigilance regulations require healthcare professionals to report adverse drug reactions (ADRs) and ensure drug safety monitoring.

    - Professionals must stay updated on drug safety guidelines, reporting requirements, and participate in pharmacovigilance activities.

    - Implications include ADR reporting, conducting signal detection and risk-benefit assessments, and implementing risk minimization strategies.

These evolving regulatory frameworks necessitate healthcare professionals to stay updated on new requirements, adapt their practices, and maintain compliance to ensure patient safety, data privacy, and regulatory adherence. Professionals may need to undergo training, establish effective documentation and reporting processes, and collaborate with regulatory bodies to navigate the changing regulatory landscape effectively.

Strategies For Adapting To Future Changes And Challenges

Adapting to future changes and challenges in the healthcare industry requires proactive strategies and a forward-thinking approach. Here are some strategies for healthcare professionals to adapt effectively (Figure 9.1):

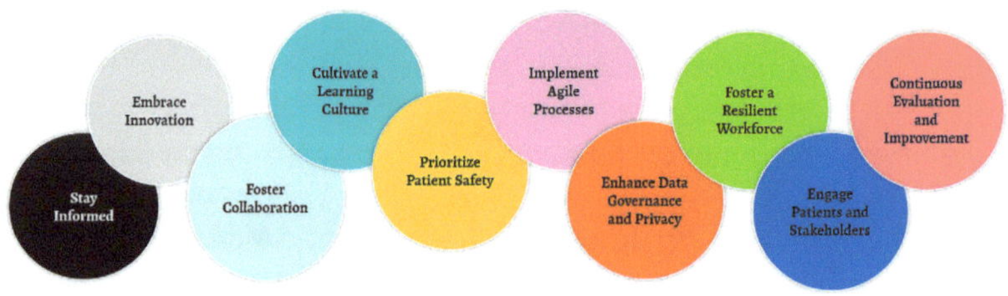

▲ **Figure 9.1**: Strategies for Adapting to Future Changes and Challenges

1. **Stay Informed:** Stay updated with the latest industry trends, regulatory changes, and emerging technologies through continuous education, attending conferences, participating in webinars, and subscribing to relevant publications. Being well-informed enables professionals to anticipate changes and plan accordingly.

2. **Embrace Innovation:** Embrace technological advancements and innovative solutions that can improve healthcare delivery, patient outcomes, and operational efficiency. Embracing telemedicine, digital health tools, and data analytics can enhance risk management, patient engagement, and decision-making processes.

3. **Foster Collaboration:** Collaborate with colleagues, industry experts, and regulatory bodies to share knowledge, exchange best practices, and navigate regulatory changes. Building strong networks and partnerships can help healthcare professionals stay adaptable and learn from others' experiences.

4. **Cultivate a Learning Culture:** Foster a culture of continuous learning and professional development within healthcare organizations. Encourage employees to pursue training, certifications, and educational opportunities to acquire new skills and stay updated with evolving industry practices.

5. **Prioritize Patient Safety:** Maintain a strong focus on patient safety in all aspects of healthcare delivery. Implement robust risk management practices, adhere to regulatory requirements, and actively seek patient feedback to identify areas for improvement and ensure patient-centered care.

6. **Implement Agile Processes:** Embrace agile methodologies and processes to adapt quickly to changes, optimize workflows, and respond to emerging challenges. Agile principles, such as iterative planning, continuous improvement, and flexibility, can enable healthcare professionals to navigate uncertainties effectively.

7. **Enhance Data Governance and Privacy:** Strengthen data governance practices to ensure the privacy, security, and integrity of patient information. Implement robust data protection measures, comply with relevant data privacy regulations, and establish policies for responsible data use and sharing.

8. **Foster a Resilient Workforce:** Invest in the well-being and professional development of healthcare professionals. Provide resources for stress management, promote work-life balance, and offer training programs to enhance resilience and adaptability in the face of change.

9. **Engage Patients and Stakeholders:** Involve patients, caregivers, and other stakeholders in decision-making processes, risk assessments, and quality improvement initiatives. Their insights and perspectives can provide valuable input for adapting to future challenges and improving healthcare outcomes.

10. **Continuous Evaluation and Improvement:** Regularly evaluate existing processes, policies, and practices to identify areas for improvement. Implement a culture of continuous quality improvement, conduct regular audits, and collect feedback from patients and staff to drive ongoing enhancements.

By implementing these strategies, healthcare professionals can navigate future changes and challenges effectively, promote innovation, and deliver high-quality care in an evolving healthcare landscape.

Implementation Roadmap

In this chapter, we present an implementation roadmap to guide healthcare professionals in the successful adoption and integration of risk-based quality management practices based on ISO 13485 and EU MDR. The roadmap provides a structured approach for implementing key components of risk-based quality management, ensuring compliance with regulatory requirements, and driving continuous improvement within healthcare organizations.

Developing A Comprehensive Roadmap For Implementing Risk-based Quality Management

Developing a comprehensive roadmap for implementing risk-based quality management requires careful planning and consideration of various factors. Here's an example of a detailed roadmap that can guide healthcare professionals in the implementation process (Figure 10.1):

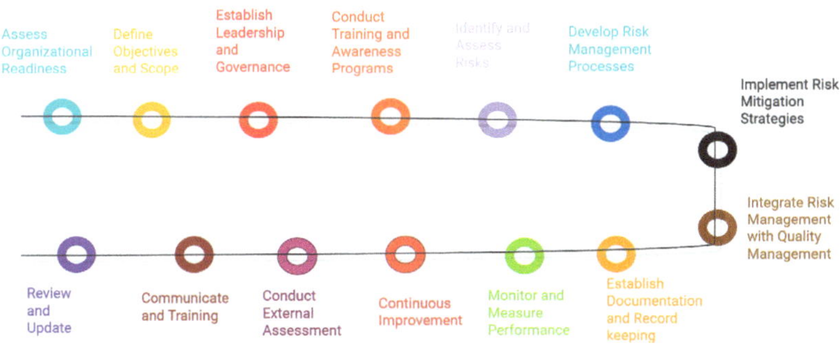

▲ **Figure 10.1**: Roadmap Implementing Risk-based Quality Management

1. **Assess Organizational Readiness:**

   - Conduct a thorough assessment of the organization's current quality management practices, risk management processes, and regulatory compliance status.

   - Identify gaps, strengths, and areas for improvement in relation to risk-based quality management.

2. **Define Objectives and Scope:**

   - Clearly define the objectives of the risk-based quality management implementation, considering regulatory requirements, patient safety goals, and organizational priorities.

   - Determine the scope of the implementation, including the departments, processes, and systems that will be impacted.

3. **Establish Leadership and Governance:**

   - Appoint a dedicated risk management team and designate responsible leaders who will oversee and guide the implementation process.

   - Develop a governance structure to ensure accountability, clear decision-making processes, and effective communication.

4. **Conduct Training and Awareness Programs:**

   - Provide comprehensive training programs on risk management principles, ISO 13485, EU MDR, and other relevant standards and regulations.

   - Raise awareness among employees about the importance of risk-based quality management and their roles in the implementation.

5. **Identify and Assess Risks:**

   - Conduct a comprehensive risk assessment across the organization to identify potential risks and their potential impact on patient safety and business operations.

   - Prioritize risks based on severity, probability, and detectability to determine areas of focus for risk mitigation efforts.

6. **Develop Risk Management Processes:**

-   Establish standardized risk management processes and procedures that align with ISO 14971 and other applicable regulations.

-   Define the roles and responsibilities of individuals involved in risk management activities.

7. **Implement Risk Mitigation Strategies:**

-   Develop and implement risk mitigation strategies and action plans to address identified risks.

-   Integrate risk controls into existing processes, systems, and workflows to minimize or eliminate potential hazards.

8. **Integrate Risk Management with Quality Management:**

-   Align risk management processes with existing quality management systems, such as document control, corrective and preventive actions, and audits.

-   Ensure seamless integration and collaboration between risk management and quality management functions.

9. **Establish Documentation and Recordkeeping:**

-   Develop a comprehensive documentation system to capture risk management activities, including risk assessments, mitigation plans, and decision-making processes.

-   Implement robust recordkeeping practices to ensure traceability, accountability, and compliance with regulatory requirements.

10. **Monitor and Measure Performance:**

-   Establish key performance indicators (KPIs) to measure the effectiveness of risk-based quality management processes.

-   Regularly monitor and evaluate the performance of risk management activities, conduct internal audits, and track progress towards established objectives.

11. Continuously Improve:

- Foster a culture of continuous improvement by regularly reviewing and updating risk management processes and practices.

- Collect feedback from stakeholders, conduct lessons learned sessions, and implement necessary changes to enhance risk-based quality management.

12. Conduct External Assessments:

- Engage external auditors or regulatory bodies to assess compliance with ISO 13485, EU MDR, and other relevant standards.

- Use assessment findings to identify areas for further improvement and ensure ongoing compliance.

13. Communicate and Train:

- Maintain ongoing communication with employees, stakeholders, and regulatory bodies to keep them informed about the progress and benefits of the risk-based quality management implementation.

- Provide regular training and refresher programs to ensure continued adherence to risk management practices.

14. Review and Update:

- Periodically review the effectiveness of the implemented risk-based quality management system and make necessary updates based on changes in regulations, industry standards, and organizational needs.

By following this comprehensive roadmap, healthcare professionals can systematically implement risk-based quality management practices and create a culture of continuous improvement and patient safety within their organizations.

Project Planning And Management Considerations

When implementing risk-based quality management in healthcare, project planning and management play a crucial role in ensuring a successful and efficient implementation process. Here are some considerations for project planning and management (Table 10.1):

1. **Define Project Objectives:** Clearly define the objectives of the risk-based quality management implementation, including specific outcomes and deliverables. This will provide a clear direction for the project team and stakeholders.

2. **Develop a Project Plan:** Create a comprehensive project plan that outlines the tasks, timelines, and dependencies involved in the implementation. Identify key milestones and establish a realistic timeline for completing each phase of the project.

3. **Allocate Resources:** Determine the necessary resources for the project, including human resources, budget, technology, and tools. Ensure that the project team has the required skills and expertise to execute the implementation effectively.

4. **Stakeholder Engagement:** Identify the key stakeholders, including executives, department heads, frontline staff, and regulatory bodies. Engage them early in the process to gain their support, input, and involvement. Regularly communicate project updates and progress to stakeholders.

5. **Risk Identification and Management:** Conduct a thorough risk assessment to identify potential risks and develop mitigation strategies. Assign responsibilities for risk management activities and ensure that risks are regularly reviewed and addressed throughout the project.

6. **Project Team Collaboration:** Foster a collaborative environment among the project team members. Encourage open communication, information sharing, and cross-functional collaboration to ensure that all aspects of the implementation are addressed effectively.

7. **Change Management:** Recognize that implementing risk-based quality management may require organizational and cultural changes. Develop a change management plan to address resistance, communicate the benefits of the new approach, and provide training and support to facilitate a smooth transition.

8. **Monitor and Evaluate:** Establish mechanisms to monitor the progress of the project and regularly evaluate its effectiveness. Use key performance indicators (KPIs) to measure project success and make adjustments as necessary.

9. **Document and Share Best Practices:** Throughout the project, document best practices, lessons learned, and success stories. This documentation will serve as a valuable resource for future projects and help create a culture of continuous improvement.

10. **Project Closure and Evaluation:** Once the implementation is complete, conduct a comprehensive evaluation of the project outcomes, lessons learned, and areas for improvement. Share the results with stakeholders and use them to inform future initiatives.

By considering these project planning and management considerations, healthcare professionals can effectively plan, execute, and monitor the implementation of risk-based quality management, leading to successful outcomes and improved patient safety.

▼ **Table 10.1**: Resource and Responsibility

Resource	Responsibility
Project Manager	Overall project management and coordination
Risk Manager	Risk assessment and management
Quality Manager	Integration with quality management system
Training Coordinator	Training and awareness programs development
Documentation Lead	Documentation system development and maintenance
IT Support	Technology infrastructure setup and support
Department Heads	Provide input and support implementation efforts
Executive Sponsor	Provide support, resources, and strategic guidance
Internal Auditor	Monitor project progress and evaluate effectiveness
Stakeholders	Engage in project activities and provide input

Stakeholder Engagement And Change Management Strategies

Stakeholder engagement and change management strategies are crucial aspects of implementing risk-based quality management in healthcare. Effectively engaging stakeholders and managing change can help ensure successful adoption and acceptance of the new approach. Here are some strategies for stakeholder engagement and change management:

1. **Identify Stakeholders:** Identify all relevant stakeholders who will be impacted by the implementation of risk-based quality management. This may include executives, department heads, frontline staff, regulatory bodies, patients, and other relevant parties.

2. **Understand Stakeholder Needs:** Gain a thorough understanding of each stakeholder's needs, concerns, and expectations regarding the implementation. Conduct surveys, interviews, or focus groups to gather feedback and insights.

3. **Communication Plan:** Develop a comprehensive communication plan to keep stakeholders informed and engaged throughout the implementation process. Provide regular updates, share progress reports, and address any concerns or questions raised by stakeholders.

4. **Executive Sponsorship:** Secure executive sponsorship to demonstrate leadership commitment and support for the implementation. Engage executives in championing the change and communicating its importance to the organization.

5. **Training and Education:** Provide comprehensive training and education programs to stakeholders to ensure they understand the principles and benefits of risk-based quality management. Tailor training programs to different stakeholder groups, addressing their specific roles and responsibilities.

6. **Stakeholder Involvement:** Actively involve stakeholders in the implementation process. Seek their input in decision-making, encourage their participation in working groups or committees, and incorporate their ideas and suggestions into the risk management framework.

7. **Change Agents:** Identify change agents within the organization who can advocate for the new approach and help facilitate its adoption. These individuals can act as ambassadors, guiding and supporting other stakeholders through the change process.

8. **Address Resistance:** Anticipate and address resistance to change. Provide clear and compelling reasons for the change, address concerns, and communicate the benefits of risk-based quality management. Offer support and resources to stakeholders who may need assistance in adapting to the new approach.

9. **Continuous Engagement:** Maintain ongoing engagement with stakeholders even after the initial implementation. Seek their feedback on the effectiveness of the risk-based quality management system, address any emerging issues, and foster a culture of continuous improvement.

10. **Celebrate Success:** Recognize and celebrate milestones and successes throughout the implementation journey. Highlight the positive impact of risk-based quality management on patient safety, operational efficiency, and regulatory compliance.

By implementing these stakeholder engagement and change management strategies, healthcare organizations can foster a supportive environment, gain buy-in from stakeholders, and successfully navigate the transition to risk-based quality management.

Monitoring And Evaluating The Effectiveness Of Risk Management Initiatives

Monitoring and evaluating the effectiveness of risk management initiatives is crucial to ensure ongoing improvement and compliance in healthcare organizations. Here are some key steps and considerations for monitoring and evaluating the effectiveness of risk management initiatives (Table 10.2):

1. **Establish Key Performance Indicators (KPIs):** Define specific KPIs that align with the goals and objectives of the risk management initiatives. These KPIs can include metrics related to incident rates, risk reduction, compliance, and patient safety.

2. **Data Collection and Analysis:** Implement systems and processes to collect relevant data for monitoring and evaluation. This can include incident reporting systems, audits, inspections, and feedback mechanisms. Analyze the collected data to identify trends, patterns, and areas for improvement.

3. **Regular Risk Assessments:** Conduct regular risk assessments to identify new or emerging risks and evaluate the effectiveness of existing risk controls. This helps ensure that risk management efforts remain up to date and aligned with changing circumstances.

4. **Compliance Audits:** Perform regular compliance audits to assess adherence to regulatory requirements and internal policies. This helps identify any gaps or non-compliance issues that need to be addressed.

5. **Incident Management and Reporting:** Implement a robust incident management system to capture and investigate incidents. Analyze incident reports to identify root causes and determine if existing risk controls are effective in preventing or mitigating risks.

6. **Stakeholder Feedback:** Seek feedback from stakeholders, including staff, patients, and regulatory bodies, to assess their perceptions of the effectiveness of risk management initiatives. Conduct surveys, focus groups, or interviews to gather qualitative insights.

7. **Review and Improvement Process:** Establish a structured review process to evaluate the effectiveness of risk management initiatives. This can include regular management reviews, internal or external audits, and continuous improvement cycles to address identified areas for enhancement.

8. **Benchmarking:** Compare risk management performance against industry standards, best practices, or similar healthcare organizations to identify areas where improvements can be made. Benchmarking helps provide context and identify areas of excellence or opportunities for improvement.

9. **Training and Education Evaluation:** Assess the effectiveness of training and education programs related to risk management. Monitor staff competency levels, knowledge retention, and application of risk management principles in their day-to-day activities.

10. **Reporting and Communication:** Communicate the findings of monitoring and evaluation activities to relevant stakeholders. This includes sharing reports, performance dashboards, and improvement recommendations to drive accountability and transparency.

By implementing a comprehensive monitoring and evaluation framework, healthcare organizations can continuously assess the effectiveness of their risk management initiatives, identify areas for improvement, and take proactive measures to enhance patient safety, compliance, and overall quality of care.

CONCLUSION

In conclusion, "Risk-Based Quality Management: A Practical Guide for Healthcare Professionals based on ISO 13485 and EU MDR" provides a comprehensive and practical resource for healthcare professionals seeking to implement effective risk-based quality management in their organizations. Throughout the book, we have explored the foundations of risk-based quality management, delved into the requirements of ISO 13485 and EU MDR, and discussed various strategies, tools, and techniques for integrating risk management into existing quality management systems.

The book has emphasized the importance of risk-based approaches in healthcare, considering the dynamic nature of the industry and the criticality of patient safety. It has provided insights into identifying and categorizing risks, conducting risk assessments, and prioritizing risks based on severity and probability. Moreover, it has highlighted the significance of risk documentation, traceability, and compliance in meeting regulatory requirements and ensuring accountability.

The integration of risk management into existing quality management systems has been a central focus, addressing the roles and responsibilities of stakeholders, developing risk management procedures and workflows, and establishing a culture of continuous improvement. The book has emphasized the value of stakeholder engagement, change management, and data-driven insights for enhancing risk management practices and driving organizational goals.

Furthermore, the book has explored compliance excellence, risk mitigation techniques, and post-market surveillance, shedding light on areas such as process controls, validation protocols, adverse event reporting, and supplier qualification and control. Real-world case studies and practical examples have showcased successful risk-based quality management implementations, enabling readers to learn from the experiences of healthcare organizations.

The provided tools, templates, and checklists offer practical resources for customization and application in specific healthcare settings, facilitating the implementation of risk-based quality management. The book has also highlighted the importance of continuous improvement, lessons learned, and future considerations, including emerging trends, technological advancements, and evolving regulatory frameworks.

In summary, "Risk-Based Quality Management" equips healthcare professionals with the knowledge, strategies, and resources necessary to establish effective risk-based quality management systems. By embracing these principles and practices, healthcare organizations can enhance patient safety, ensure compliance, and drive continuous improvement in the ever-changing landscape of healthcare. This book serves as a valuable guide and reference for healthcare professionals committed to delivering high-quality care while effectively managing risks.

Recap Of Key Concepts And Takeaways

Throughout the book, "Risk-Based Quality Management: A Practical Guide for Healthcare Professionals based on ISO 13485 and EU MDR," we have covered a range of key concepts and takeaways. Here is a recap of some of the essential points:

1. **Risk-Based Quality Management:** Risk-based approaches are crucial in healthcare to proactively identify, assess, and mitigate risks to patient safety and product quality. It involves integrating risk management into quality management systems to ensure effective decision-making and compliance.

2. **ISO 13485:** ISO 13485 is an internationally recognized standard for quality management systems specific to the medical device industry. It provides guidelines and requirements for organizations to establish and maintain a comprehensive quality management system.

3. **EU MDR:** The European Union Medical Device Regulation (EU MDR) is a regulatory framework that sets out the requirements for the safety and performance of medical devices in the European Union. It introduces stricter regulations to enhance patient safety and product quality.

4. **Risk Assessment:** Risk assessment is a systematic process of identifying, analyzing, and evaluating risks associated with medical devices or healthcare processes. It helps prioritize risks based on their severity and probability, enabling effective risk management strategies.

5. **Compliance:** Compliance with regulatory requirements is essential for healthcare organizations. It involves adhering to applicable laws, regulations, and standards to ensure patient safety, product quality, and legal obligations.

6. **Stakeholder Engagement:** Engaging stakeholders, including employees, patients, regulators, and suppliers, is crucial for effective risk management. Stakeholders should be involved in risk identification, assessment, and decision-making processes to foster a culture of collaboration and accountability.

7. **Continuous Improvement:** Continuous improvement is a fundamental principle of risk-based quality management. It involves regularly evaluating and enhancing processes, systems, and practices to drive ongoing improvement in patient safety, product quality, and organizational performance.

8. **Monitoring and Evaluation:** Monitoring and evaluating the effectiveness of risk management initiatives is vital to track progress, identify areas for improvement, and ensure compliance. Key performance indicators (KPIs), data collection, incident management, and stakeholder feedback play important roles in this process.

9. **Case Studies:** Real-world case studies and practical examples provide valuable insights into successful risk-based quality management implementations. They offer lessons learned, best practices, and practical guidance for healthcare professionals.

10. **Tools and Templates:** The book provides downloadable tools, templates, and checklists to assist healthcare professionals in implementing risk-based quality management. These resources can be customized and applied to specific healthcare organizations.

11. **Future Considerations:** The book explores emerging trends, technological advancements, and evolving regulatory frameworks that impact risk-based quality management. It emphasizes the need for healthcare professionals to stay informed and adaptable to future changes and challenges.

Overall, the book emphasizes the importance of risk-based quality management in healthcare, offering practical guidance, tools, and real-world examples to help healthcare professionals implement effective risk management practices. By embracing these concepts and takeaways, healthcare organizations can enhance patient safety, ensure compliance, and drive continuous improvement in the dynamic healthcare landscape.

Final Thoughts On Risk-Based Quality Management In Healthcare

In conclusion, Risk-Based Quality Management in healthcare is essential for ensuring patient safety, product quality, and regulatory compliance. This comprehensive approach enables healthcare professionals to identify, assess, mitigate, and monitor risks effectively, ultimately improving the overall quality of care provided.

By embracing the principles and practices outlined in this book, healthcare organizations can establish robust risk management systems that align with ISO 13485, EU MDR, and other regulatory frameworks. It empowers healthcare professionals to manage risks proactively, make informed decisions, and drive continuous improvement.

Throughout the book, we have explored the foundations of risk-based quality management, discussed the requirements of ISO 13485 and EU MDR, and provided practical strategies, tools, and templates for implementation. Real-world case studies and examples have showcased successful risk management implementations, offering valuable insights and lessons learned.

Key concepts such as risk assessment, compliance, stakeholder engagement, continuous improvement, and monitoring and evaluation have been emphasized. The book has also highlighted emerging trends, technological advancements, and evolving regulatory frameworks, urging healthcare professionals to stay adaptable and proactive in addressing future challenges.

Ultimately, Risk-Based Quality Management requires a collaborative and proactive approach from all stakeholders involved in healthcare. It is a continuous journey of improvement and adaptation, driven by a commitment to patient safety, product quality, and regulatory compliance.

By embracing the knowledge and practical guidance provided in this book, healthcare professionals can navigate the complex landscape of risk management, mitigate potential risks, and enhance the overall quality and safety of healthcare delivery.

Encouragement For Continued Learning And Professional Development In The Field

In risk-based quality management in healthcare, continued learning and professional development are essential for staying updated with the latest industry trends, regulations, and best practices. As the healthcare landscape continues to evolve, it is crucial for healthcare professionals to invest in their knowledge and skills to drive continuous improvement and ensure patient safety.

Continued learning not only expands your expertise but also enables you to adapt to emerging challenges and seize new opportunities. Here are a few encouraging thoughts to inspire your ongoing learning journey in this field:

1. **Embrace a Growth Mindset:** Approach learning with an open and curious mindset. Embrace challenges and view them as opportunities for growth. Recognize that there is always more to learn and explore in the dynamic field of risk-based quality management.

2. **Stay Informed:** Stay updated with the latest developments, regulations, and industry best practices. Engage in continuous education through attending conferences, workshops, webinars, and industry events. Follow reputable sources, journals, and professional associations to access valuable insights and resources.

3. **Seek Professional Certifications:** Consider pursuing professional certifications in risk management, quality management systems, or specific regulatory frameworks relevant to your role. These certifications demonstrate your commitment to excellence and provide a structured framework for developing your expertise.

4. **Network and Collaborate:** Engage with peers, industry experts, and thought leaders in the field. Join professional networks, participate in forums, and engage in discussions to share experiences, exchange knowledge, and gain valuable perspectives.

5. **Learn from Case Studies:** Real-world case studies offer practical insights and lessons learned from successful risk-based quality management implementations. Analyze these case studies to understand different approaches, challenges faced, and strategies employed by healthcare organizations.

6. **Engage in Continuous Improvement:** Continuously evaluate your own practices and processes. Seek feedback from colleagues, patients, and stakeholders to identify areas for improvement. Embrace a culture of continuous improvement by implementing feedback loops and incorporating lessons learned into your risk management practices.

7. **Mentorship and Collaboration:** Engage in mentorship opportunities to learn from experienced professionals in the field. Collaborate with colleagues and cross-functional teams to leverage their expertise and foster a culture of knowledge-sharing and collaboration.

8. **Embrace Technological Advancements:** Stay abreast of technological advancements and their impact on risk-based quality management. Explore how emerging technologies such as artificial intelligence, data analytics, and digital platforms can enhance risk assessment, monitoring, and decision-making processes.

Remember, continued learning and professional development are lifelong journeys. By investing in your knowledge and skills, you contribute to the advancement of risk-based quality management practices in healthcare. Embrace the challenges, seek opportunities for growth, and remain passionate about delivering high-quality care while mitigating risks and ensuring patient safety. Your commitment to ongoing learning will make a positive impact on both your professional development and the healthcare industry as a whole.

GLOSSARY OF TERMS

Terms	Definitions
Risk	The combination of the probability of occurrence of harm and the severity of that harm
Risk Management	The systematic application of management policies, procedures, and practices to the tasks of analyzing, evaluating, controlling, and monitoring risks.
Hazard	A potential source of harm
Risk Assessment	The overall process of risk identification risk analysis and risk evaluation
Risk Identification	The process of finding recognizing and describing risks
Risk Analysis	The process of comprehending the nature of risks and determining their level of acceptability
Risk Evaluation	The process of comparing the results of risk analysis with risk criteria to determine whether the risk and/or its magnitude is acceptable or tolerable
Risk Control	The process of implementing measures to reduce the risk to an acceptable level
Residual Risk	The risk remaining after risk control measures have been implemented
Risk Acceptance	The decision to accept risk based on a risk evaluation
Risk Management Plan	A document that outlines the approach activities and responsibilities for managing risks throughout the product life cycle
Risk Register	A document that captures and records identified risks including their description severity, likelihood and risk control measures
Risk Mitigation	The implementation of actions or measures to reduce the likelihood or severity of a risk

Contd ...

Terms	Definitions
Post-Market Surveillance	The systematic process of collecting, analyzing and monitoring information on the safety and performance of medical devices after they have been placed on the market
Non-Conformity	A deviation or failure to meet specified requirements or standards
Corrective Action	Actions taken to eliminate the causes of a detected non-conformity or other undesirable situation
Preventive Action	Actions taken to eliminate the causes of potential non-conformities or other undesirable situations
Quality Management System (QMS)	A set of policies, processes, and procedures implemented by an organization to ensure that products or services consistently meet customer and regulatory requirements.
Validation	The process of establishing documented evidence that a system or process, when operated within specified parameters, can perform effectively and consistently.
Verification	The process of evaluating a system or component to determine whether it complies with specified requirements
Risk Benefit Analysis	The process of evaluating and comparing the risks associated with a medical device against its intended benefits to determine if the benefits outweigh the risks
Hazardous Situation	A circumstance in which a medical device has the potential to cause harm
Probability	The likelihood of a specific event or outcome occurring
Severity	The degree of harm that can result from a hazardous situation or event
Risk Management File	A compilation of documents and records related to risk management activities, including risk assessments, risk control measures, and risk management reports.
Risk Management Review	A systematic evaluation of the effectiveness of risk management activities and the identification of any necessary updates or improvements
Risk Communication	The process of sharing information about risks associated with a medical device to stakeholders, such as healthcare professionals, patients, and regulatory authorities.
Risk Residual Limit	The maximum acceptable level of risk after risk control measures have been implemented

Contd ...

Terms	Definitions
Risk Monitoring	The ongoing process of tracking and evaluating the effectiveness of risk control measures and identifying any emerging risks
Adverse Event	Any untoward medical occurrence associated with the use of a medical device, including device malfunctions, injuries, or deaths.
Risk Register Update	The process of periodically reviewing and updating the risk register to reflect changes in the identified risks, their severity, likelihood, and risk control measures.
Risk Management Training	Educational programs and initiatives designed to enhance the knowledge and skills of individuals involved in risk management activities
Risk Management Team	A multidisciplinary group of individuals responsible for conducting risk management activities, including representatives from engineering, quality assurance, regulatory affairs, and clinical disciplines.
Risk Management Documentation	Written records and reports that document the risk management process, including risk assessments, risk management plans, and risk management reports.
Risk Management SOPs	Standard operating procedures that outline the step-by-step processes and instructions for conducting risk management activities in accordance with established policies and regulations

REFERENCES

Here are some references that can be used as sources of information for further reading on risk management in the medical device industry:

1. ISO 14971:2019 - Medical devices - Application of risk management to medical devices

2. Regulation (EU) 2017/745 of the European Parliament and of the Council of 5 April 2017 on medical devices

3. ISO 13485:2016 - Medical devices - Quality management systems - Requirements for regulatory purposes

4. FDA Guidance Documents (available on the U.S. Food and Drug Administration website)

5. IEC 60601-1: Medical electrical equipment - Part 1: General requirements for basic safety and essential performance

6. ISO/TR 24971:2020 - Medical devices - Guidance on the application of ISO 14971

7. FDA Quality System Regulation (QSR) 21 CFR Part 820

8. GHTF/SG3/N15:2011 - Risk management throughout the life cycle of medical devices

9. AAMI TIR45:2012 - Guidance on the use of agile practices in the development of medical device software

10. MDSAP Companion Document

11. ISO 10993: Biological evaluation of medical devices

12. ISO 11607: Packaging for terminally sterilized medical devices

13. ISO 15223-1: Medical devices - Symbols to be used with medical device labels, labeling, and information to be supplied - Part 1: General requirements

14. IEC 80001-1:2010 - Application of risk management for IT-networks incorporating medical devices - Part 1: Roles, responsibilities, and activities

15. ISO 31000:2018 - Risk management - Guidelines

16. MEDDEV 2.7/1 Rev. 4: Clinical Evaluation